The
POWER
of a Note

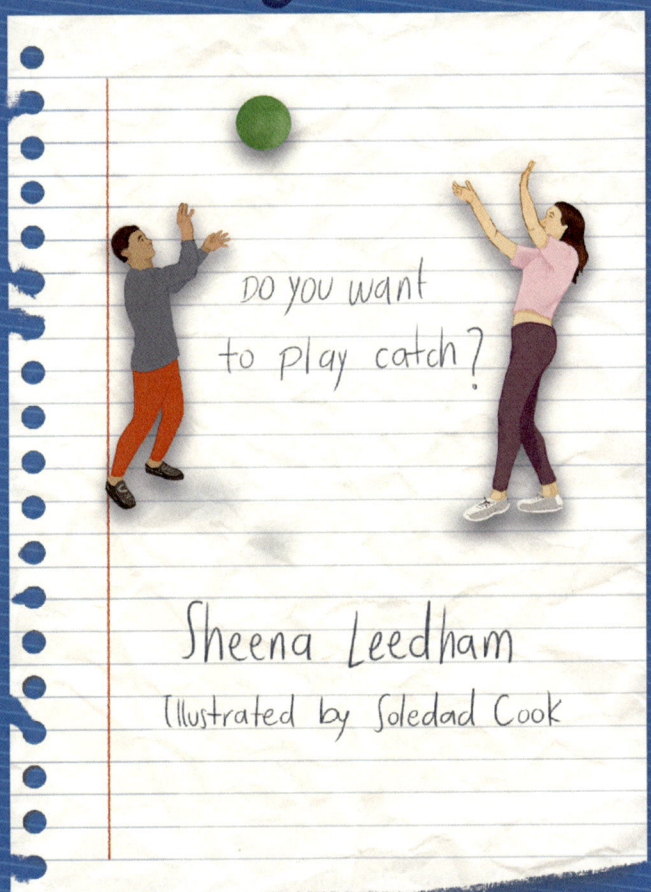

Do you want to play catch?

Sheena Leedham

Illustrated by Soledad Cook

The fitness journey of a child with autism that began with pen and paper.

CONTENTS

DEDICATION

Dedicated to the many families and clients I've been lucky to work with to sharpen my craft. To my family and friends for always supporting my passionate work to better the lives of children and young adults with autism.

FOREWORD

The story you're about to read is an accumulation of working with hundreds of children and young adults with autism. Although my formal education prepared me to be a schoolteacher in the elementary public school catering to neurotypical children in grades kindergarten through sixth, my professional experiences led me to be a facilitator of physical education for autistic children in the recreational setting. The gym serves as my schoolhouse to teach and create positive change for children and families touched by autism.

As a parent, educator, or personal trainer, use *The Power of a Note* to positively introduce exercise into a child's life touched by autism—this is what separates exercise as a weekend frustration from a lifelong journey.

Thank you for your ongoing commitment to best serve the children and young adults under your care.

HOW TO USE THIS BOOK

Based on a true story, *The Power of a Note—Storybook* takes us to a gym in London, Ohio. You'll meet a boy with autism named Blaine, who is disinterested in exercising and preoccupied with a Nintendo DS. With some observation, a pen, and a piece of paper, I'm able to switch the script. Blaine suddenly becomes curious and creative about movement and play while the DS powers down. Dave, Blaine's dad, trusts my direction and shifts from a frustrated personal trainer to a relaxed dad. With strength training being a weekly part of Blaine's development for seven years strong, this story is where and how it all began.

In *The Power of a Note—Outreach*, you'll find the benefits of exercise and training methodology serving as the foundation of Blaine's training session chunked into manageable parts. Each step references the *Storybook*, providing ample opportunity to see teachable moments in action. I encourage you to flip the pages back and forth to receive constant visual reinforcement to bridge the gap between theory and practice. Although the overall goal is to replicate my observation, communication, schedule, progression, and motivation processes for the child under your care, start small. Tweak, change, and adopt what makes sense for you and the child today. If something reads as unfamiliar and bizarre for your current training demands, don't use it, at least yet. Being aware of these programming methods, you can expect to see your role change and effectiveness flourish. As a parent, you'll be able to clearly distinguish between well-suited programming and inadequate programming when choosing a professional to join your child's network. As a professional, you'll be able to take a clearer look at your training methodology and pinpoint where you can make changes to become a better facilitator of physical education for children with autism.

Beyond *Outreach*, you'll find a sixty-minute *Schedule Sample* outlining the illustrated workout from the *Storybook*. Use this as an example of how to segment a training session into time slots, remaining cognizant of the moving parts, their order, and use of transitions.

Blaine's *Training Success* spans across seven years, and in this chapter, discover how *The Power of a Note* naturally redefines exercise for Blaine to encompass training adventures offsite and annual competition plans—to the playground, bike trail, indoor Putt-Putt, indoor trampoline park, indoor laser tag park, high school track and field, corn maze, and zoo we go!

In the final section, *Parental Feedback—Why the Note is Empowering,* Blaine's dad shares a heartfelt reflection. As a prominent figure in the strength and conditioning industry (CEO of elitefts.com—educating and outfitting the strongest athletes around the world), Dave Tate details his struggle as a father taking on a trainer role, pinpointing when and why he had to accept a change to best meet the needs of his son.

The
POWER
of a Note

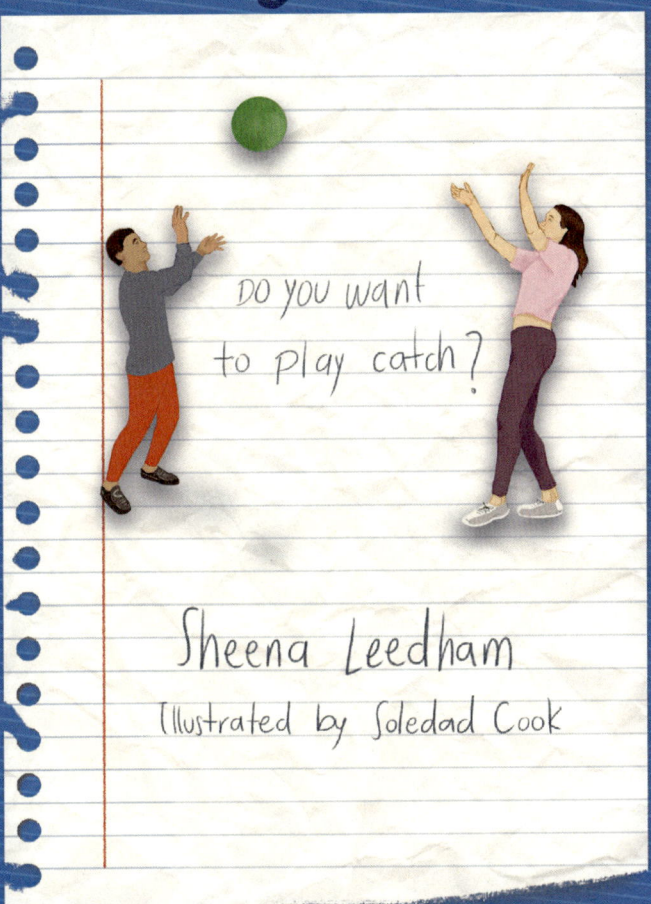

DO you want
to play catch?

Sheena Leedham

Illustrated by Soledad Cook

The fitness journey of a child with autism that began with pen and paper.

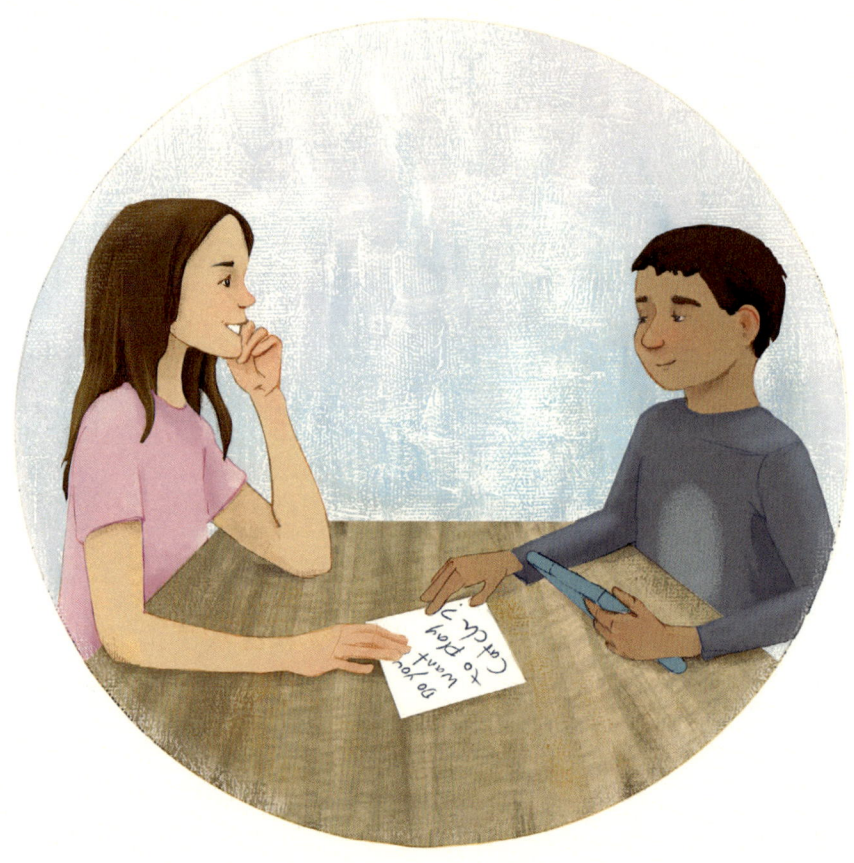

The fitness journey of a child with autism that began with pen and paper.

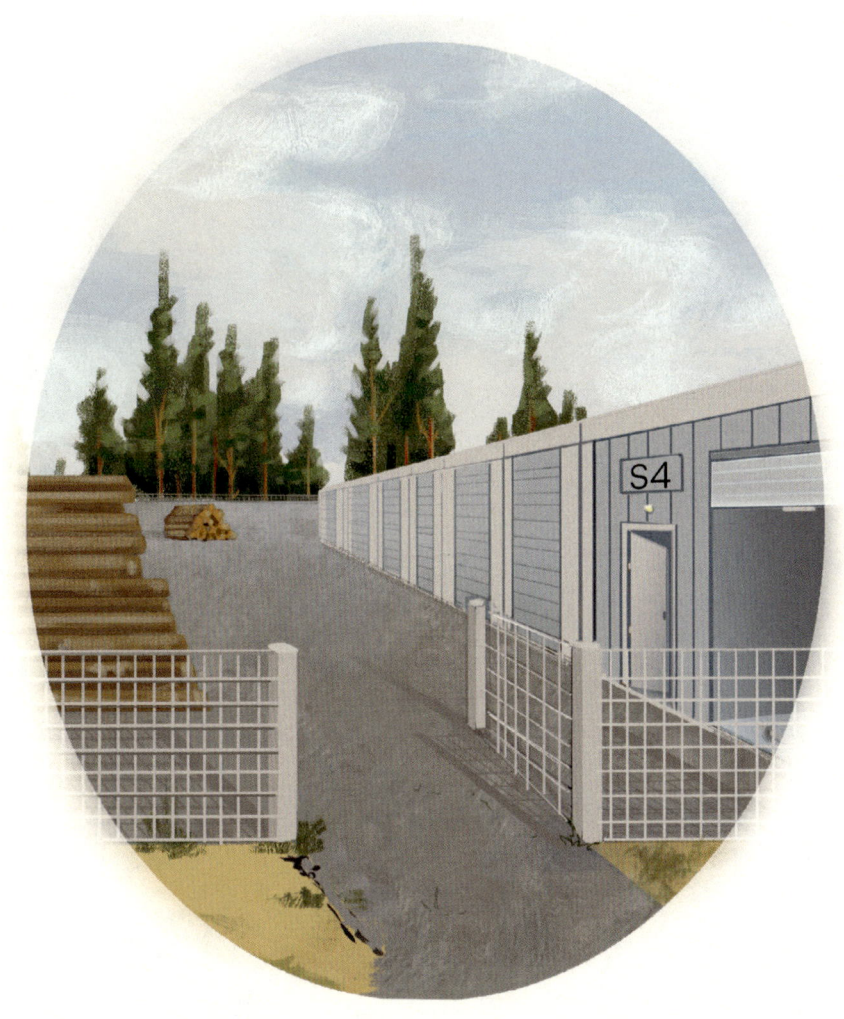

Nested in the small town of London, Ohio, before you cross the railroad tracks on Maple Street, sits a warehouse on the left. Up a crumbly cemented ramp and past the barb-wired fence, the S4 Compound shares parking lot space with a lumber yard. Outside, a no-frills structure with sturdy siding, a doorknob, and a garage door is all one can see, but inside...

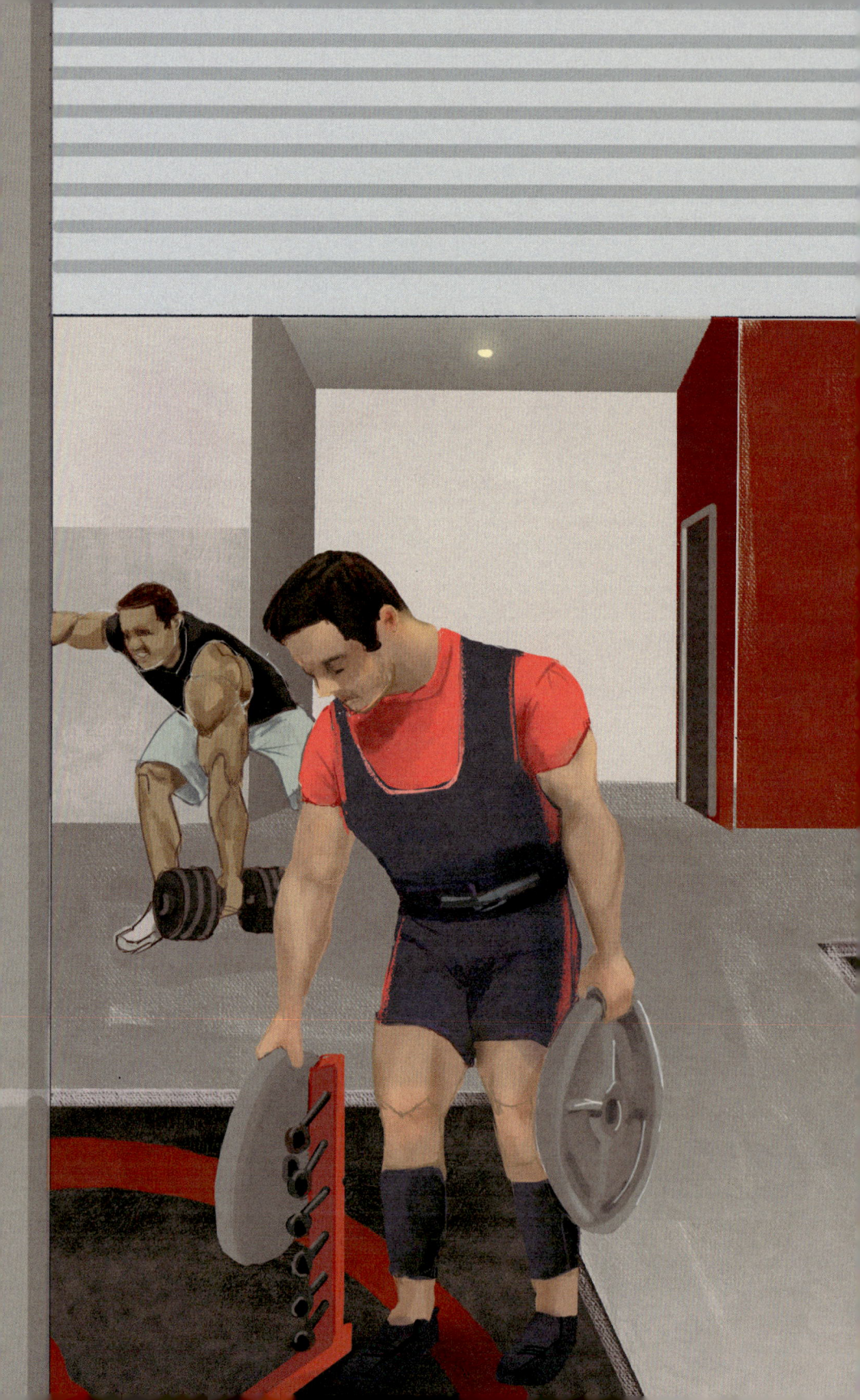

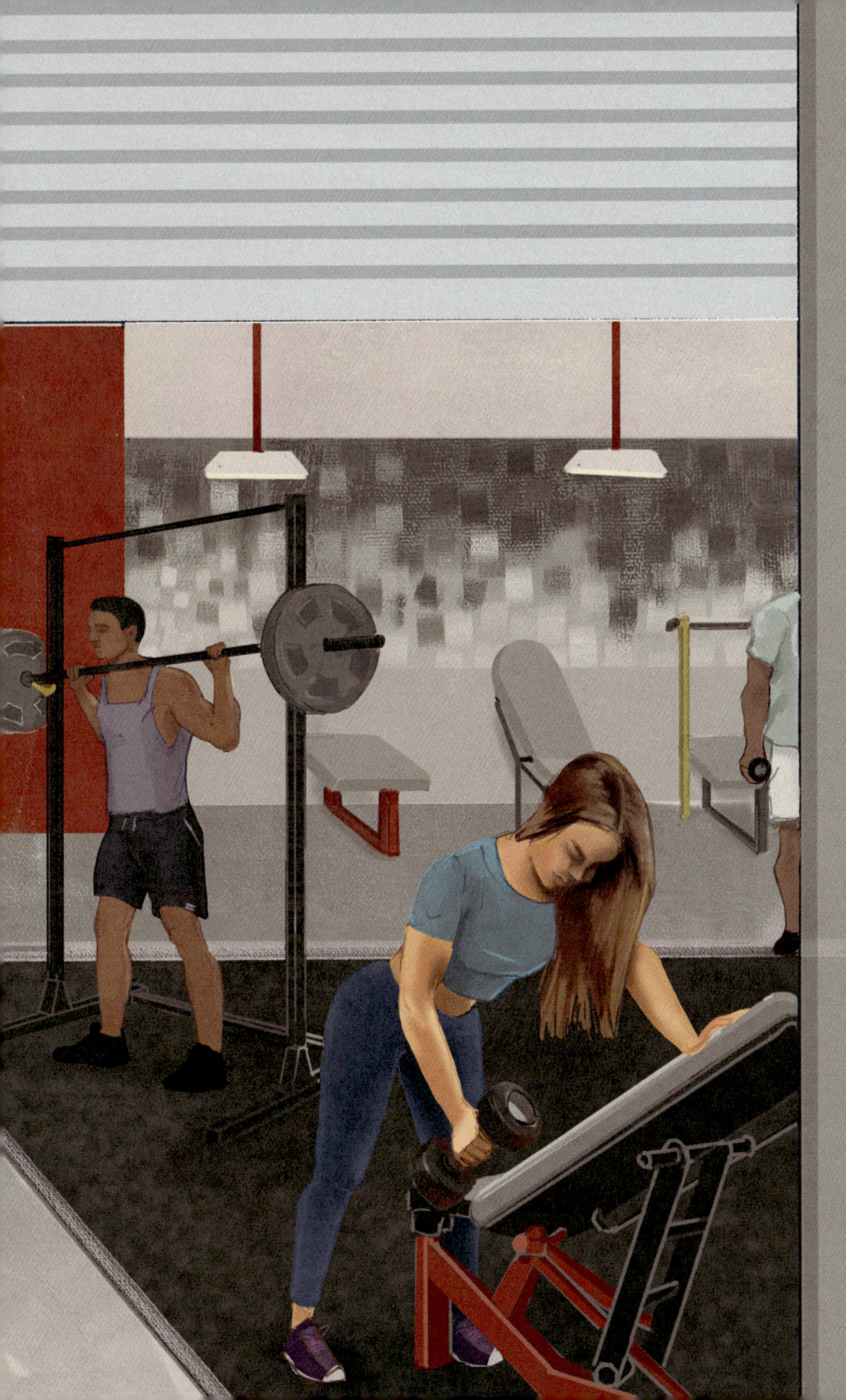

In an alarming—holy cow, I'm going to have an accident in my pants, the house is on fire, and there's a US shortage of Internet—type of way, Blaine would ask, "Are we done yet?" every two minutes. It wasn't the politest way of asking the same question over and over again.

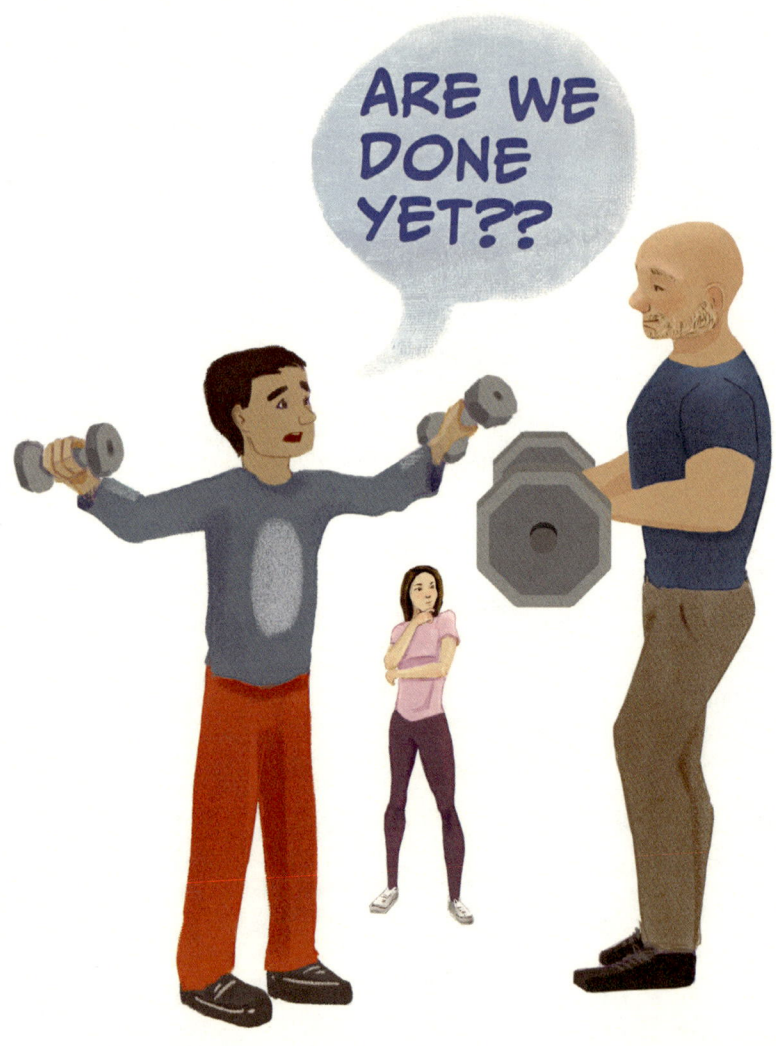

Dave, Blaine's dad, pulled out all tricks in his bag to get his son to exercise for twenty minutes. And even though Dave's the barbell whisperer in many lands, Blaine desperately anticipated hearing three words and three words only.

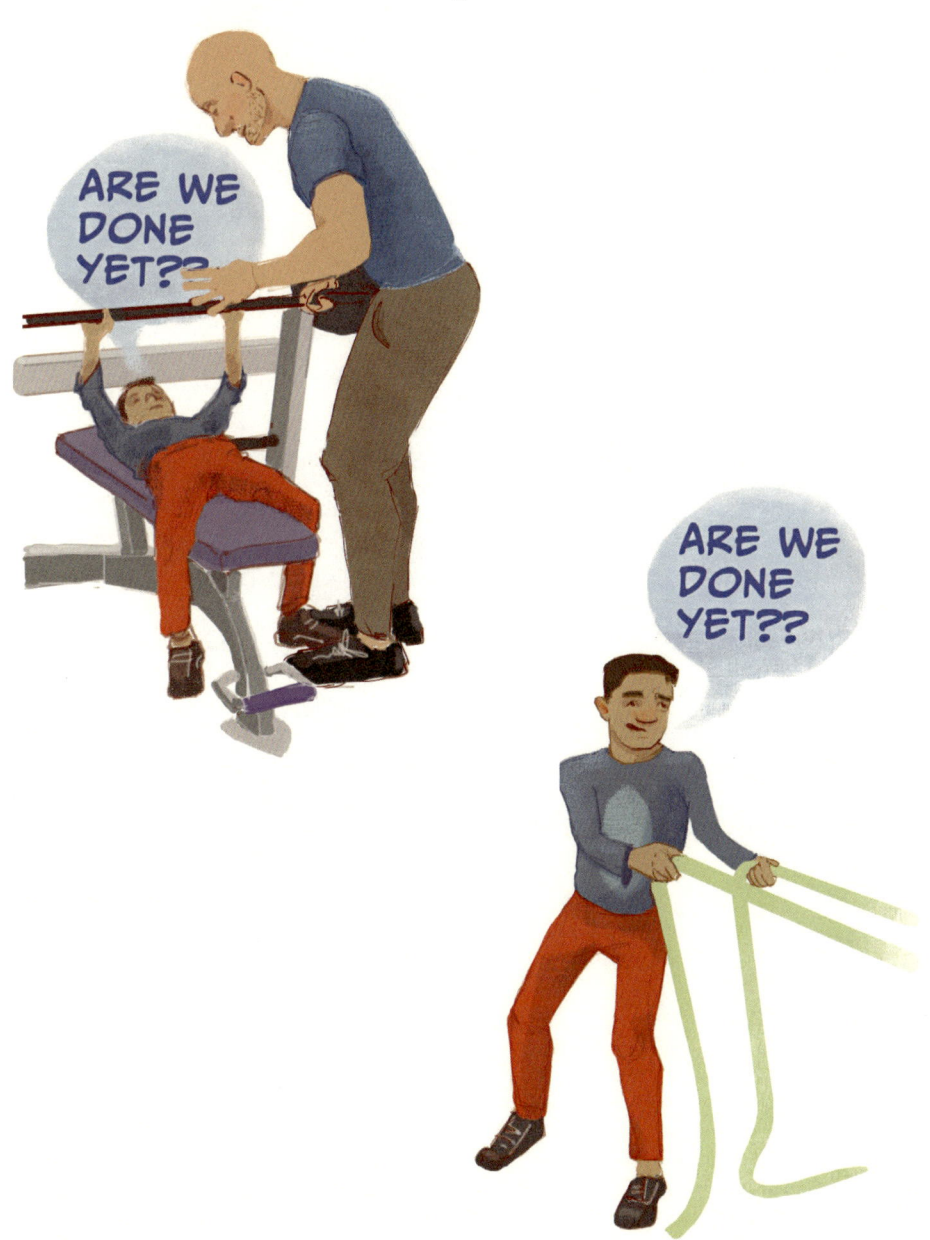

A few exercises, twenty minutes, and five gray hairs later, Dave exhaustingly said, "We are done."

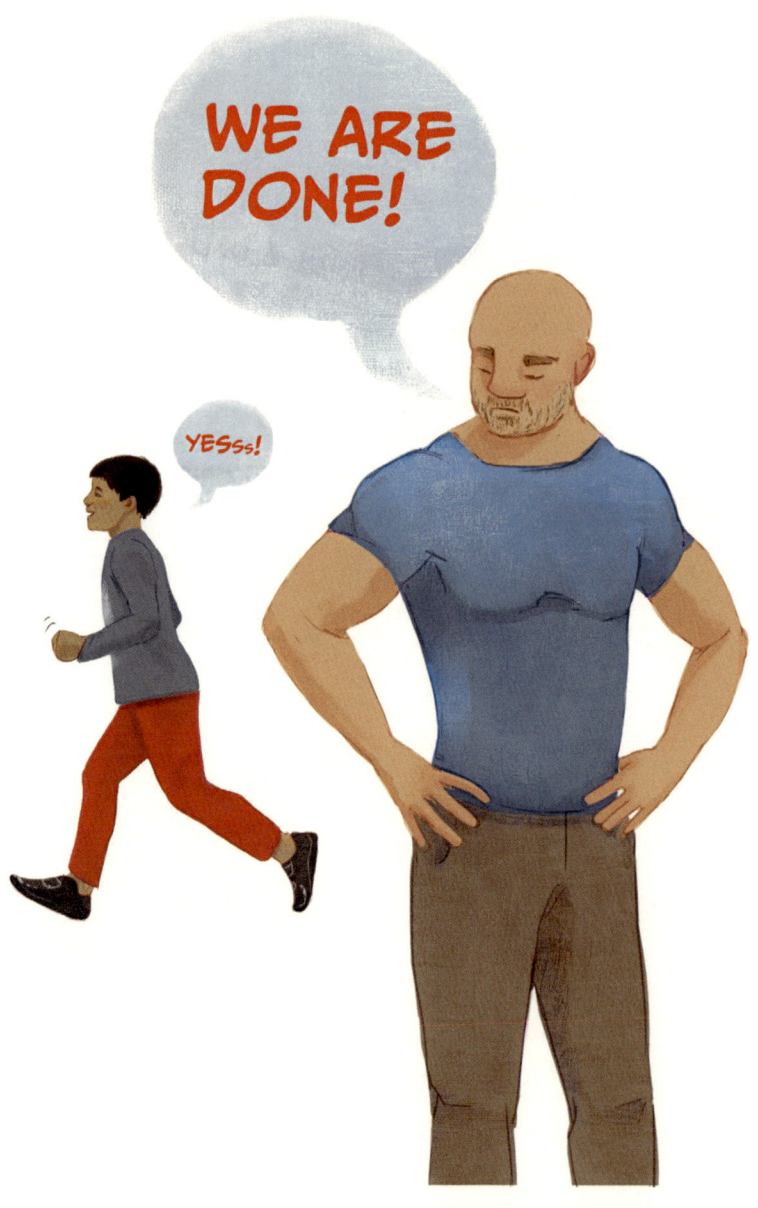

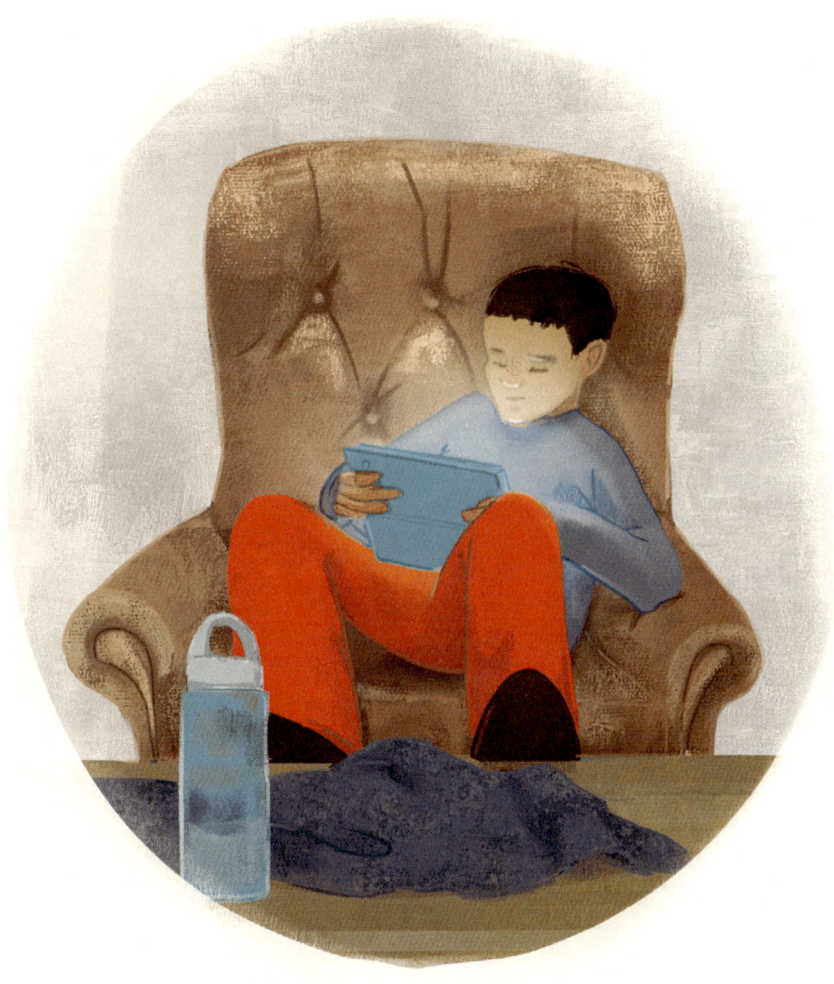

As quick as cereal with a crunch turns soggy in a bowl of milk, Blaine ran to a comfortable leather chair and took his Nintendo DS in hand.

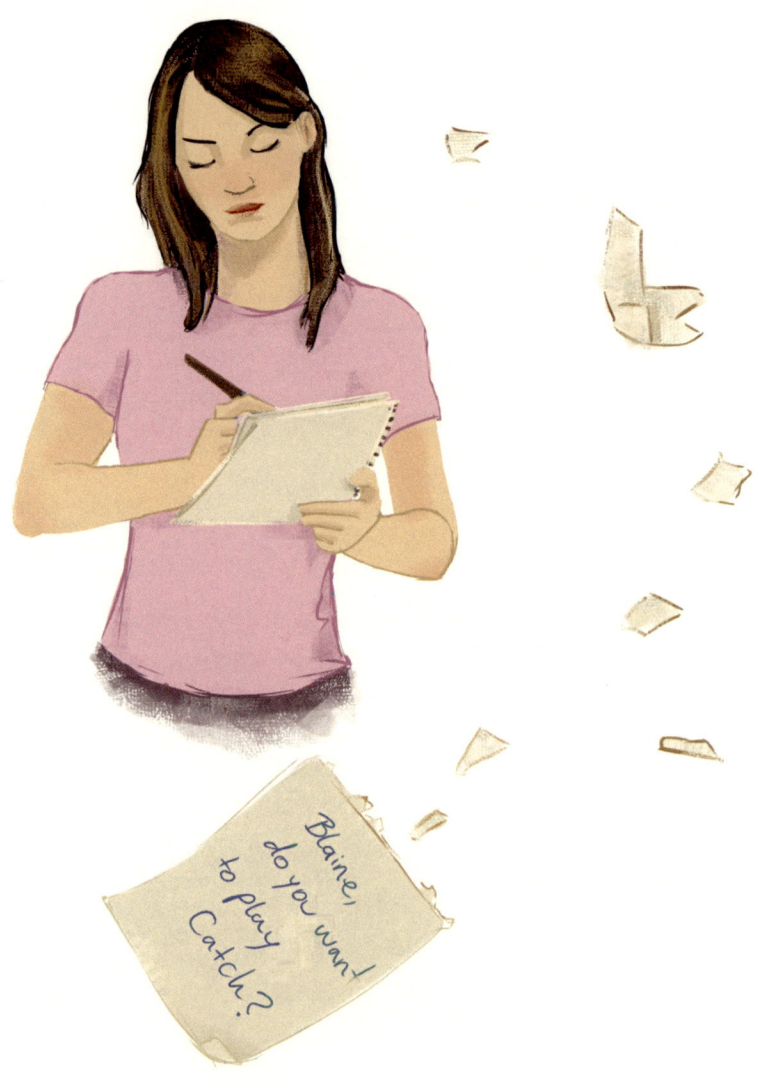

With a pen and piece of paper, I wrote, "Blaine, do you want to play catch?"

Careful enough to not sabotage his life-threatening maneuvers and earned fighting power, I slowly tugged on the paper's edge, removed the excess perforated scrap, folded it in fours, and slid the note in his direction.

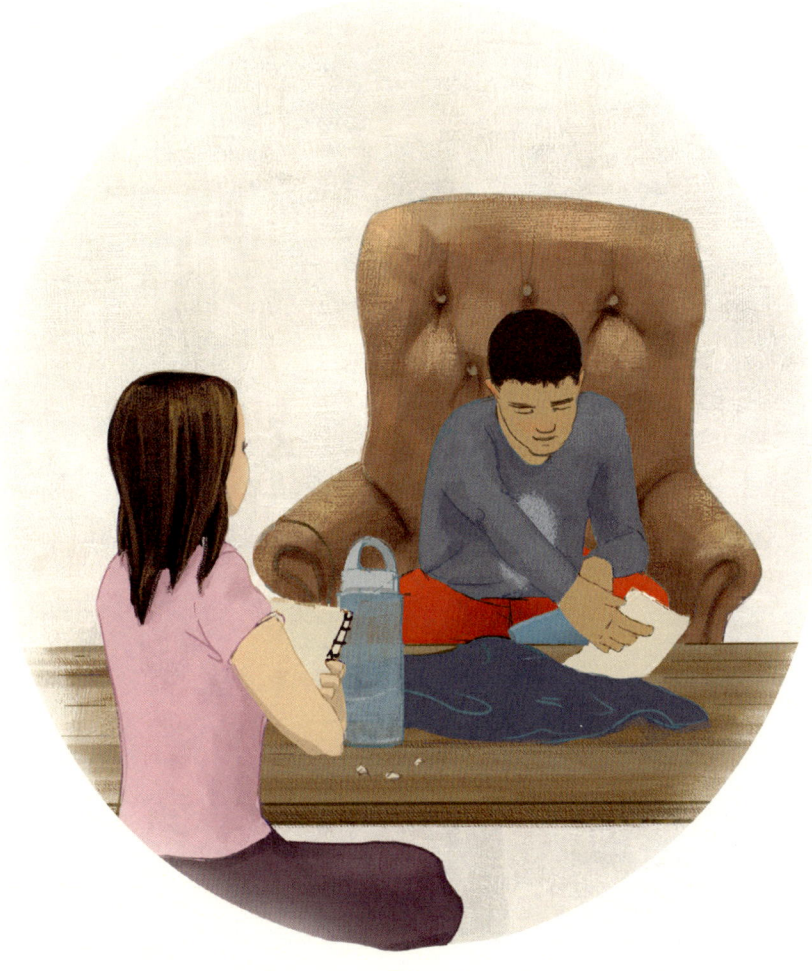

Blaine instantly paused his game, opened the folded piece of paper, and silently read the question with a half-smile.

Eyes wide open and back upright, he answered, "Give me a minute."

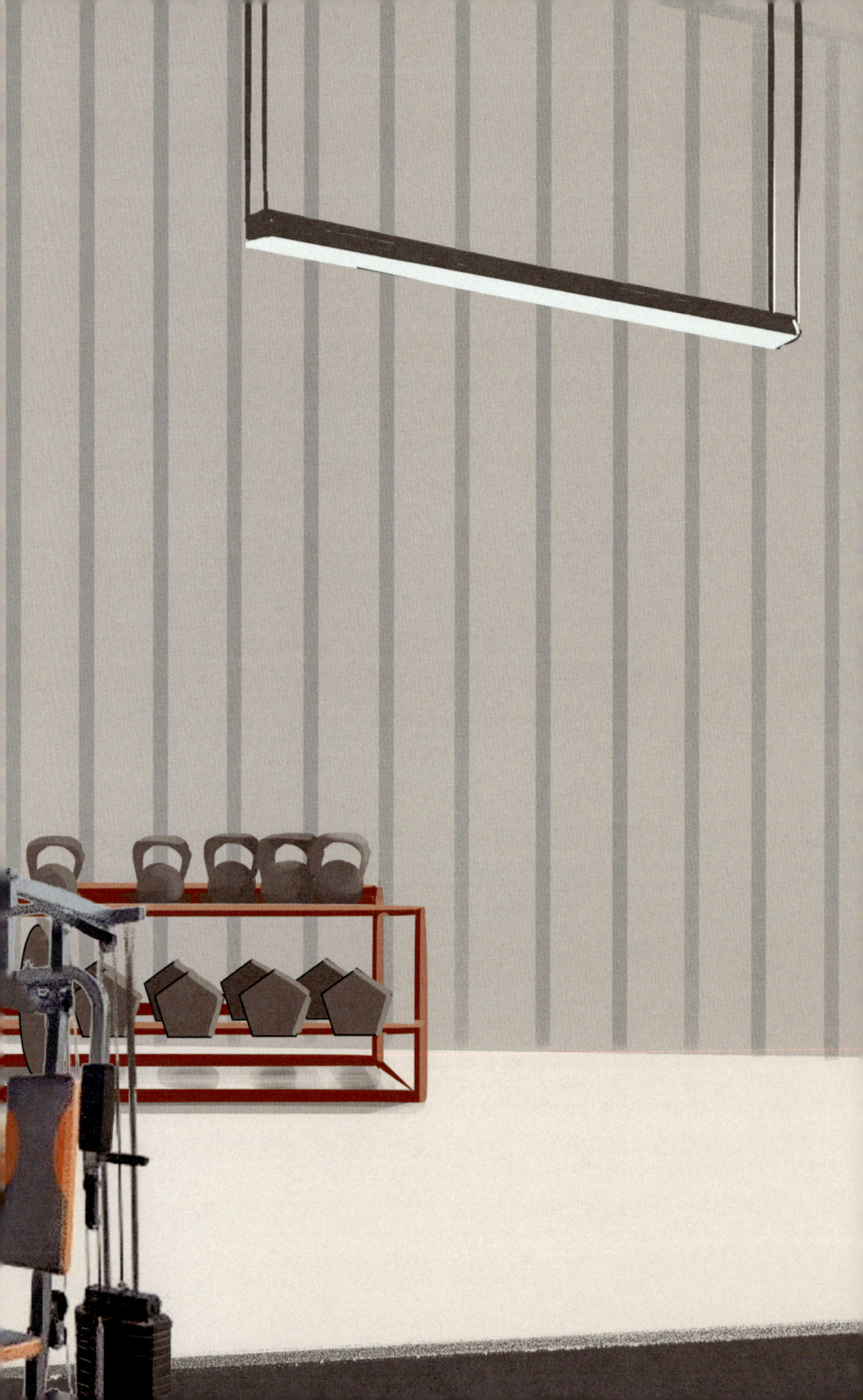

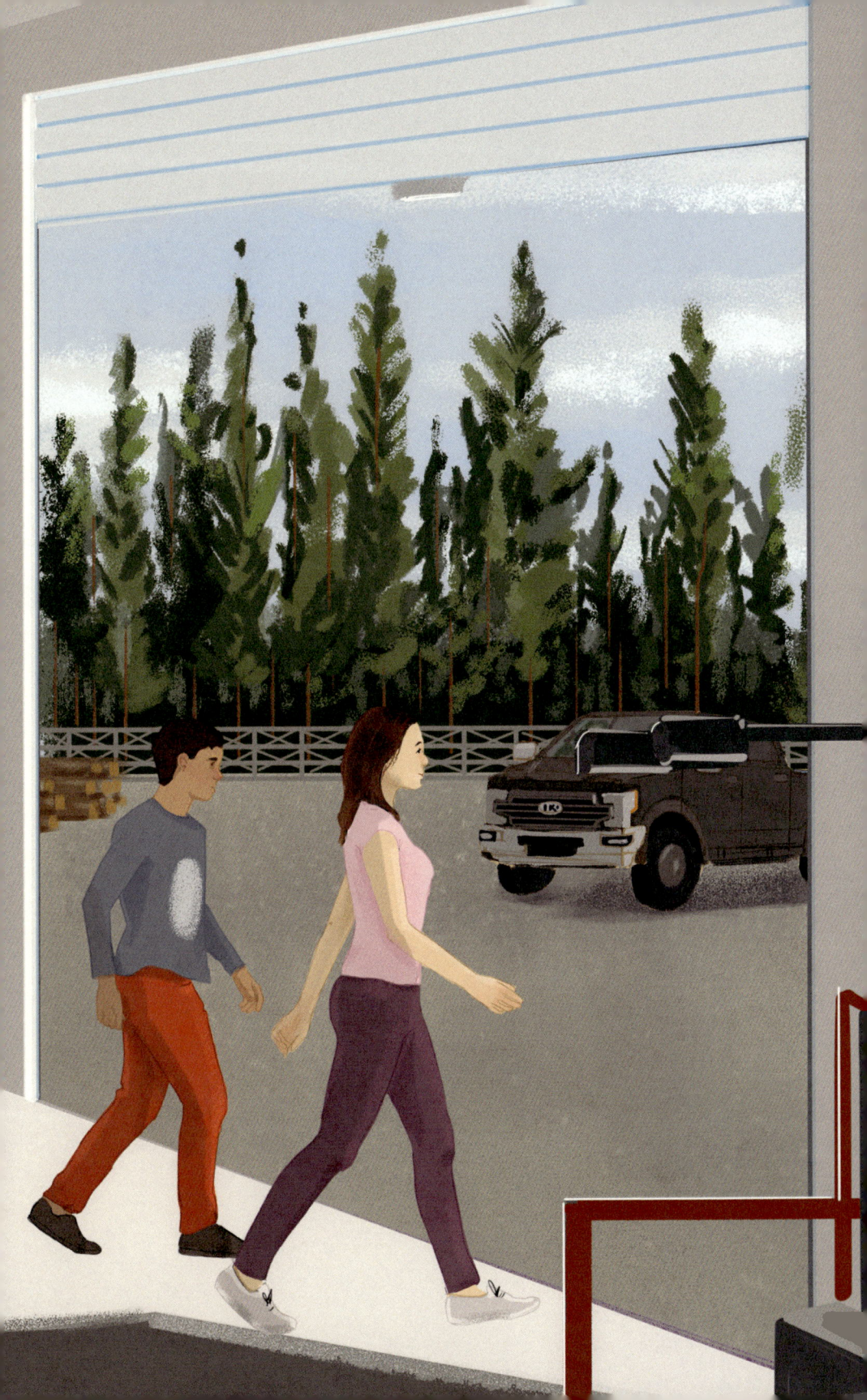

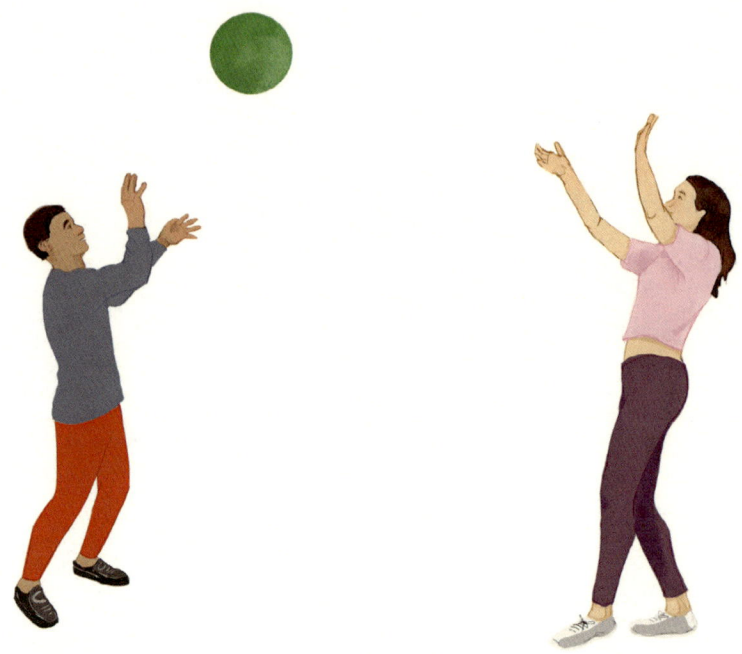

We tossed a bouncy green ball back and forth. We stepped back one foot for every complete pass until we could no longer successfully make a catch.

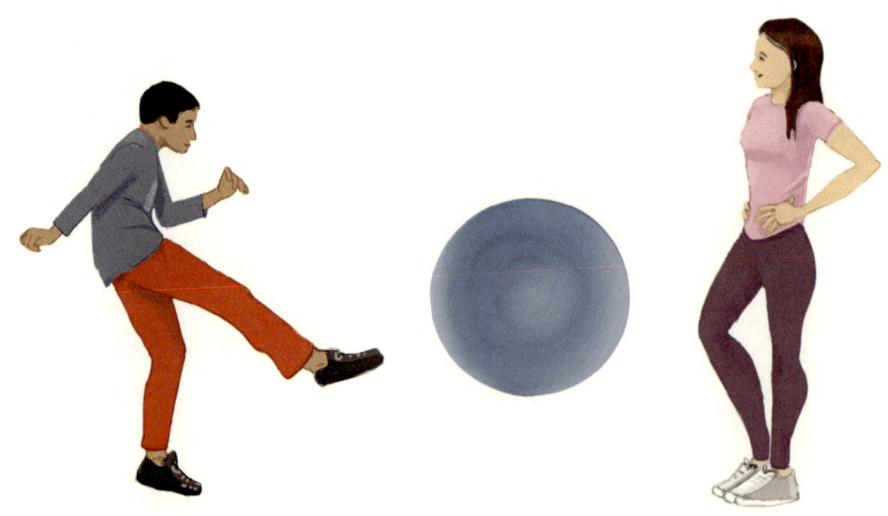

We found the largest stability ball and kicked it back and forth—five cement sliders followed by five air flyers for three rounds.

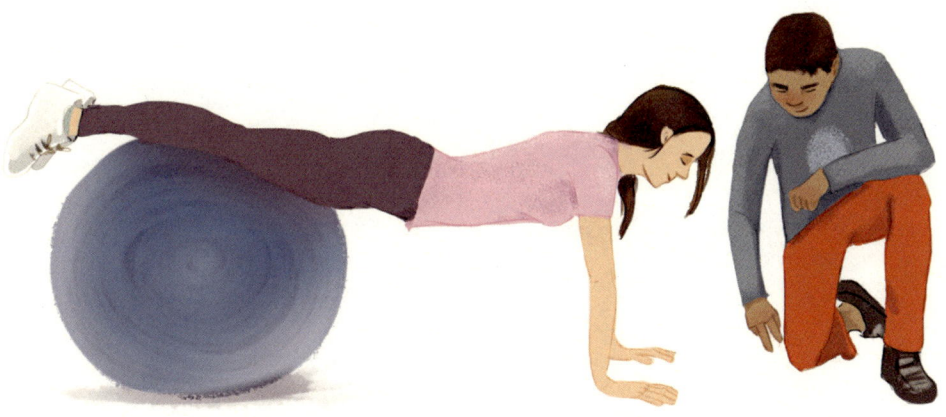

We took turns walking with our hands—four steps forward followed by four steps backward. Blaine came up with the idea to hold the end position for time—he beat my time by nine seconds.

Next, we played a game. Given two options (hide-n-seek or freeze tag), Blaine chose freeze tag—the zombie edition.

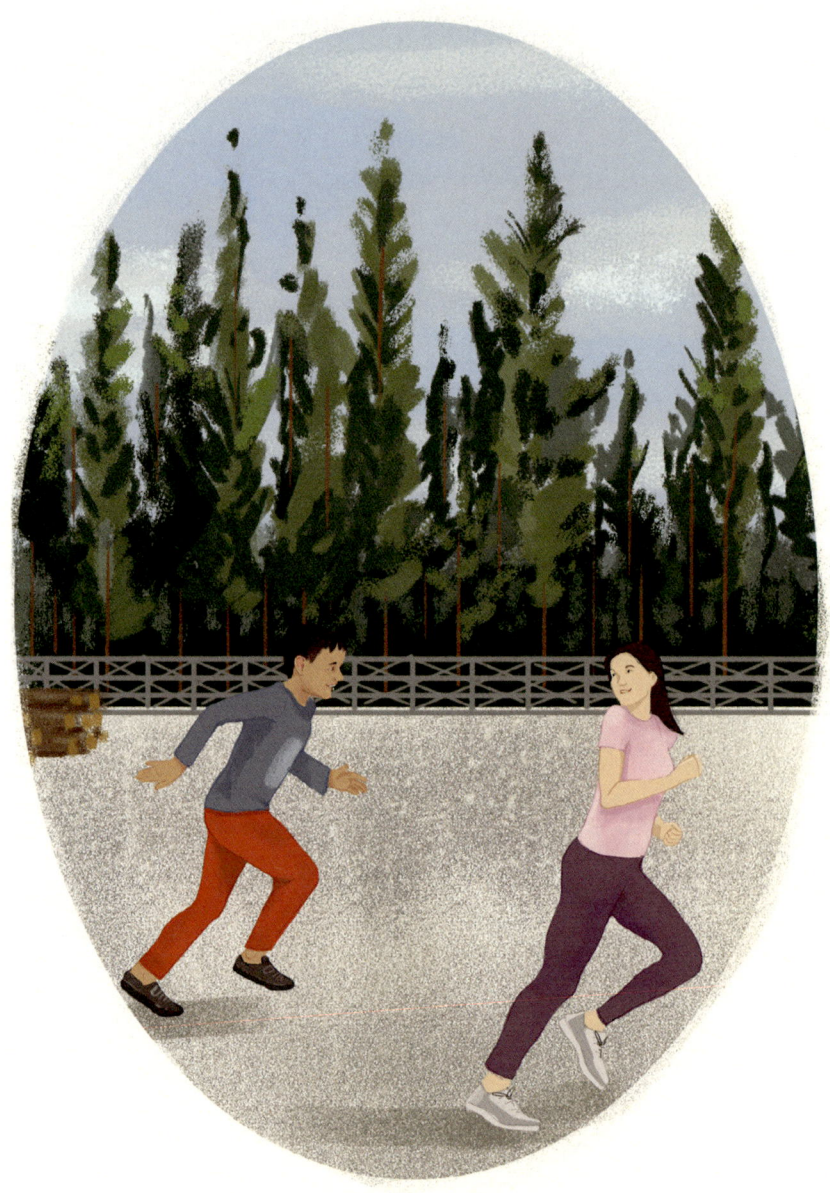

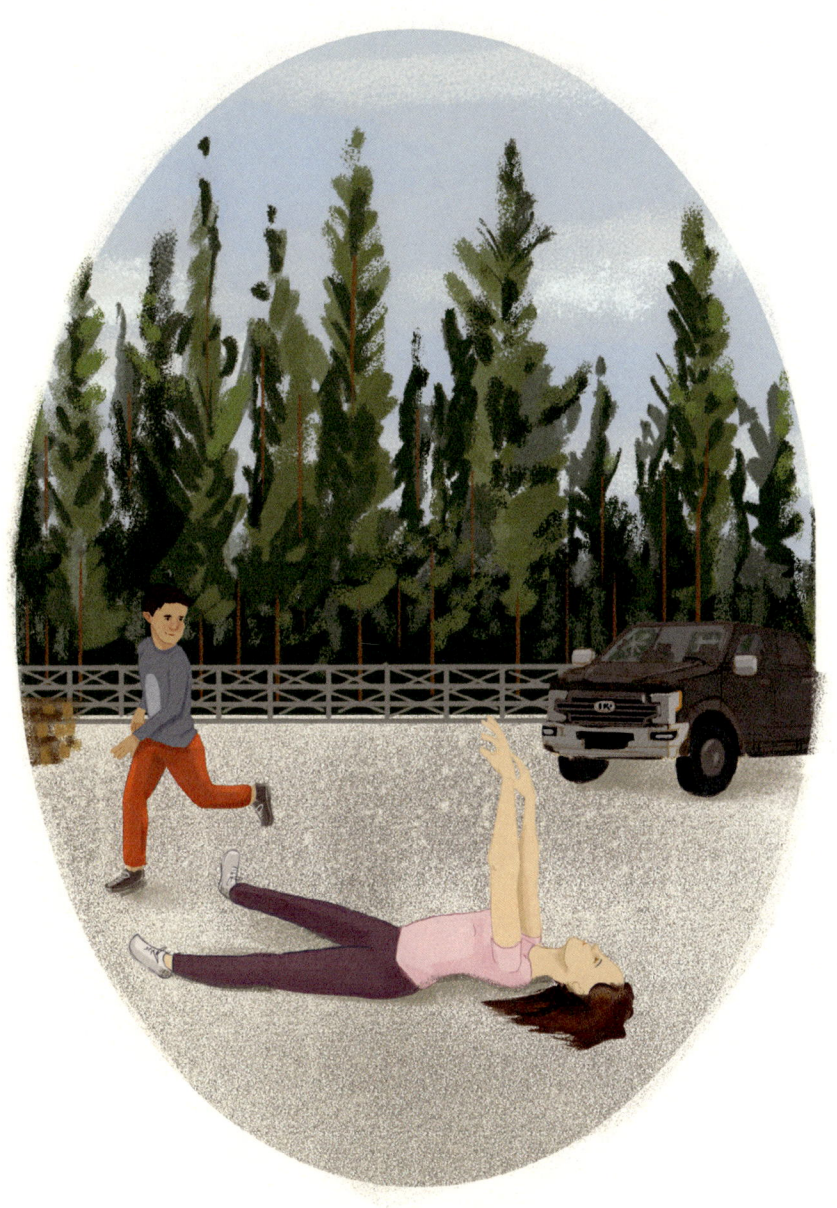

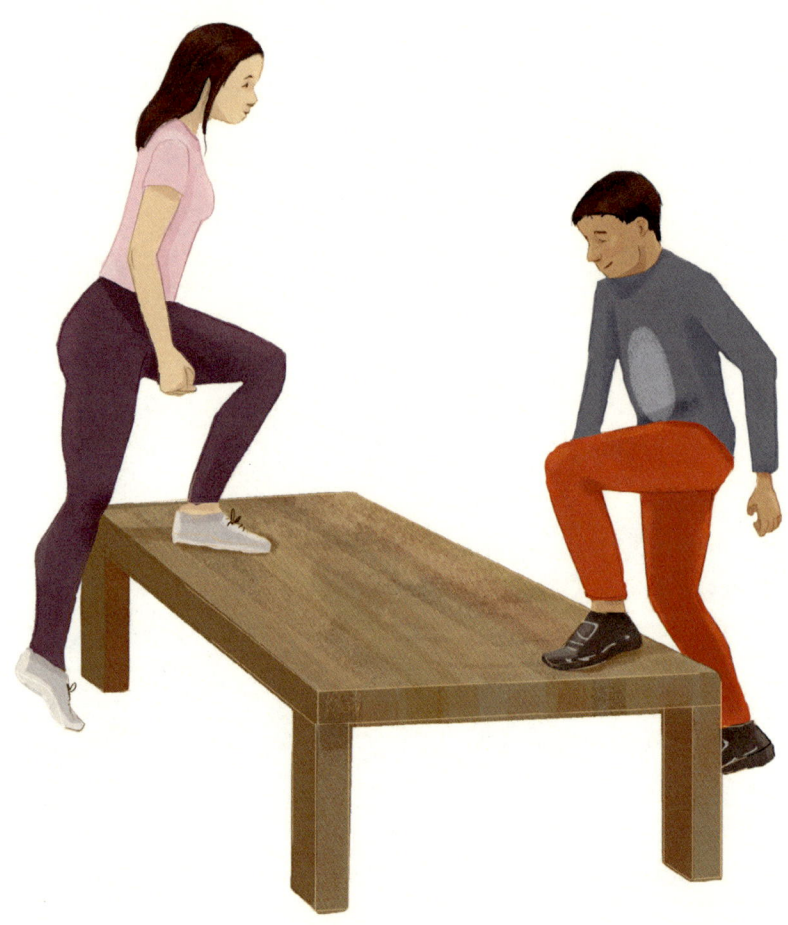

In a final and conscious attempt to make us "sweat blood," Blaine created the following obstacle course:

Table climbs × 12

360 × 12

Run to dad's truck × 1

Tap dad's truck × 5

Run back to table × 1

We raced through the course for two rounds. I won once, and Blaine won once.

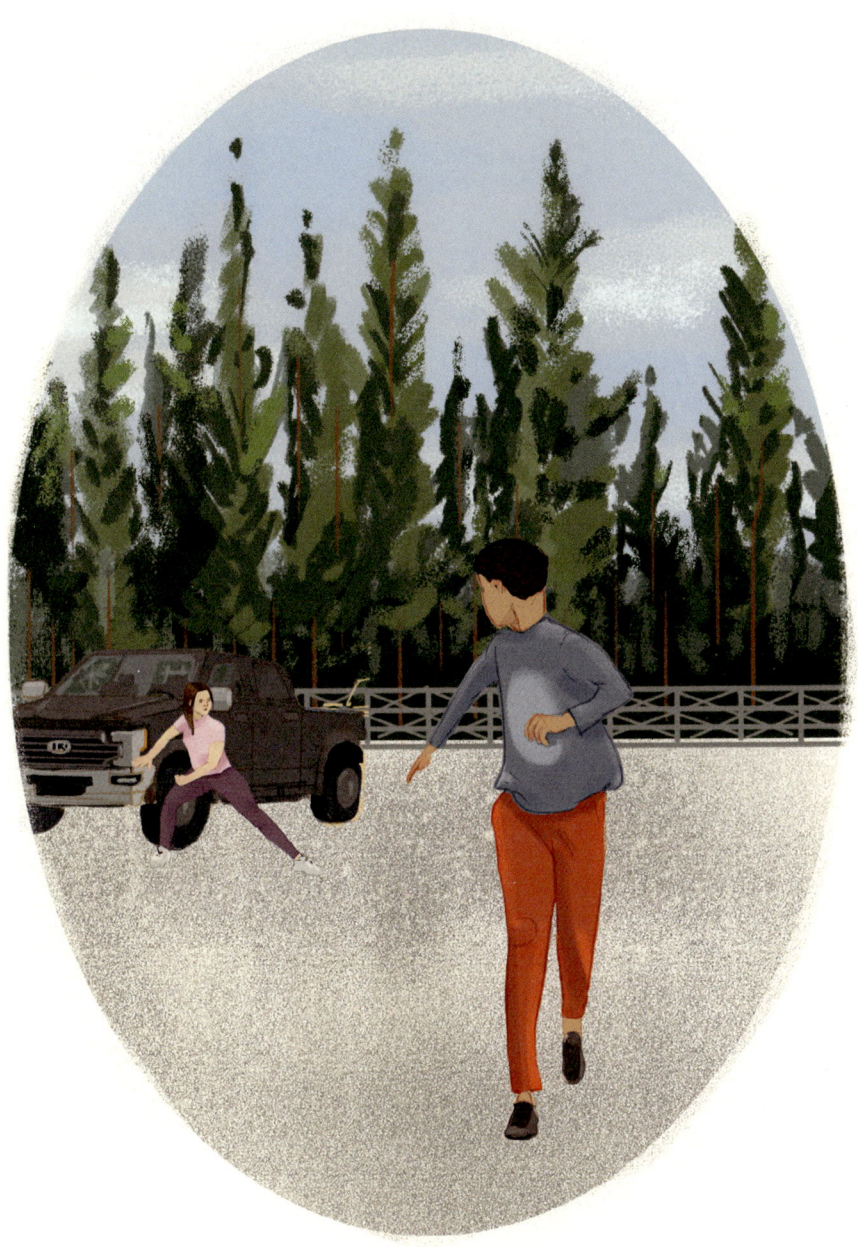

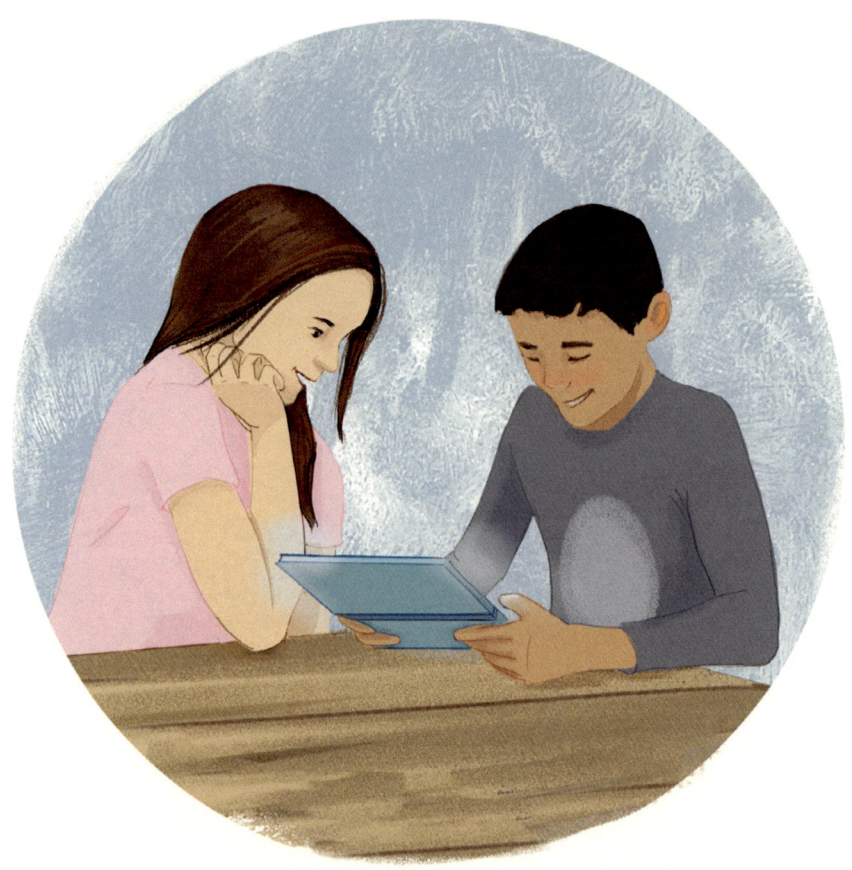

"Blaine, we should do this—gasp—every—gasp—Tuesday!"

"Yeah. I probably lost around seven pounds today," Blaine said.

For free time, Blaine excitedly ran inside the gym to grab his DS and bring it outside. In five minutes, he taught me how to start and pause the game, run forward, jump, and crouch.

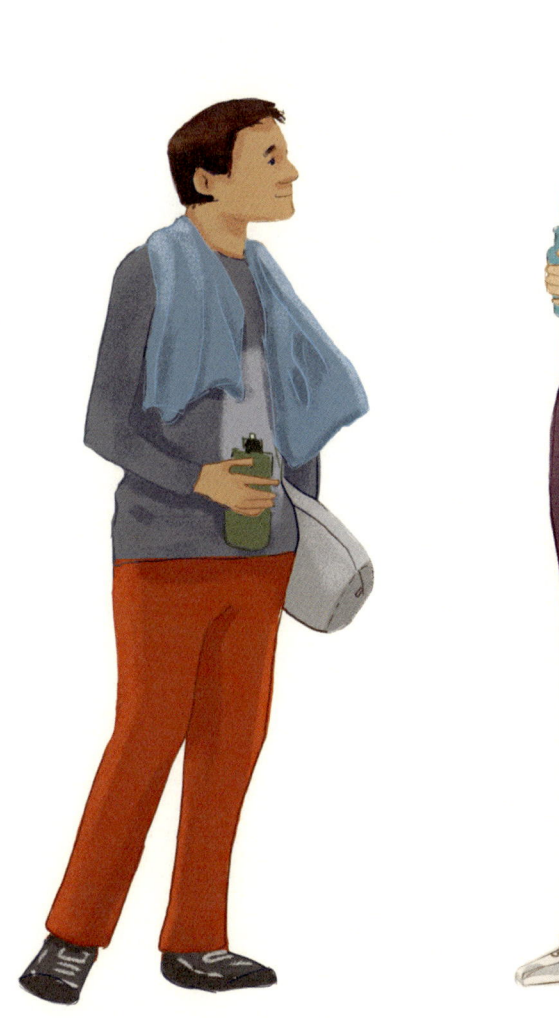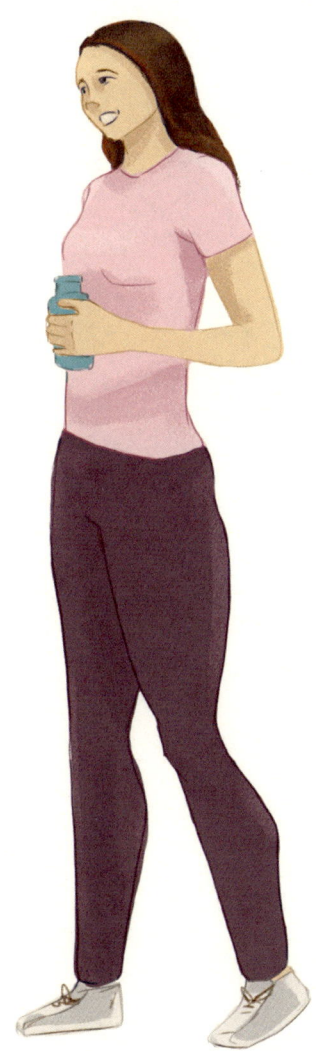

And so, our fitness journey began.

OUTREACH

Benefits of Exercise

Children with autism have been found to have low levels of physical fitness, contributing to an increase in inactivity and weight gain. Physical movement is perceived to be threatening and uncomfortable; therefore, it's easy for autistic children to overindulge in passive and consumptive behaviors like watching television and playing video games (Smith & Gouze, 2004). Dawson and Rosanoff (2009) report that more than fifty percent of children with autism are either overweight or at risk. Due to this lack of physical movement (activities like walking, running, swinging, bike riding, playing, jumping, tumbling, climbing, pushing, pulling, swimming, and sledding), the development of generic skills contributes to limited motor functioning, low motivation, difficulty in planning, and difficulty in self-monitoring.

Physical movement is a key ingredient for new learning and development. With an acknowledgment of sensitivity to stimuli (auditory, visual, and tactile), movement expands the brain's ability to form new neurological connections and gives the body newfound ability (Baniel, 2012).

Through an individualized training program, we can introduce exercise skills at a young age to promote health, fitness, and habitual activity (Drabik, 1996). When individuals with autism are consistently physically active, the benefits include alleviated stress and anxiety (Hillier et al., 2011), significantly decreased negative self-stimulating behaviors, promotion of self-esteem and positive social outcomes (Dawson & Rosanoff, 2009), and reduced risk of hypertension, obesity, and diabetes (Jacobs, 2018).

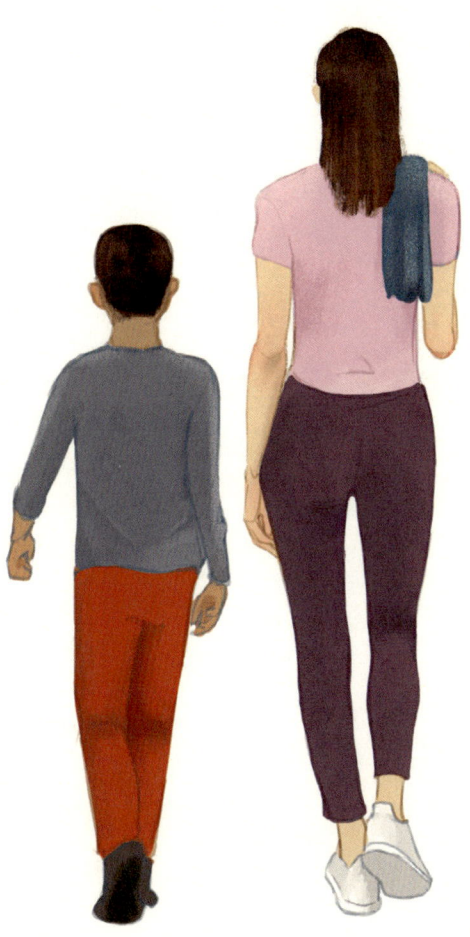

Use *The Power of a Note* to replicate my observation, communication, schedule, progression, and motivation processes for the child under your care—positively introduce exercise and make movement a lifelong journey.

STEP ONE:

OBSERVE

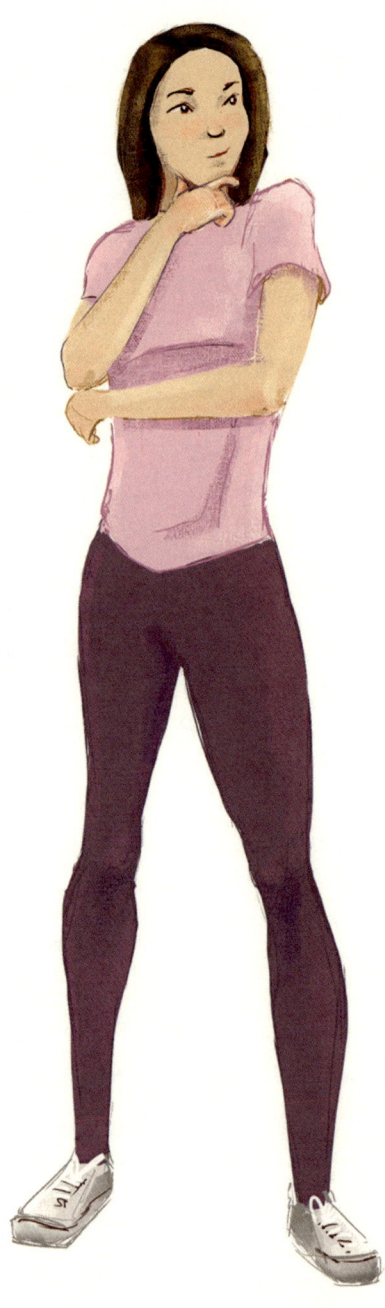

Observe the child in his or her natural environment without distraction and judgment (Baniel, 2012). Take mental and written notes. When is the child most receptive to the world around him? What are the child's needs? What is the child capable of today? What are the child's interests? What are the caregiver's expectations? Start your efforts here.

Observation Application

As I observed Blaine and his dad, Blaine was mostly receptive toward his dad when he was playful and funny. Noteworthy, Blaine needed to be entertained throughout the session and was heavily motivated by his Nintendo DS. At ten years old, Blaine needed improvement in coordination, endurance, speed, strength, flexibility, and spatial awareness.

Emotionally, Blaine perceived exercise to be strenuous, boring, and a means to an end. Although his dad did not use this session to introduce anything unfamiliar to Blaine, Dave was mindful of when and when not to correct technique. Based on my observation, I determined play would be my vehicle to get Blaine moving and reshape his negative perception of movement.

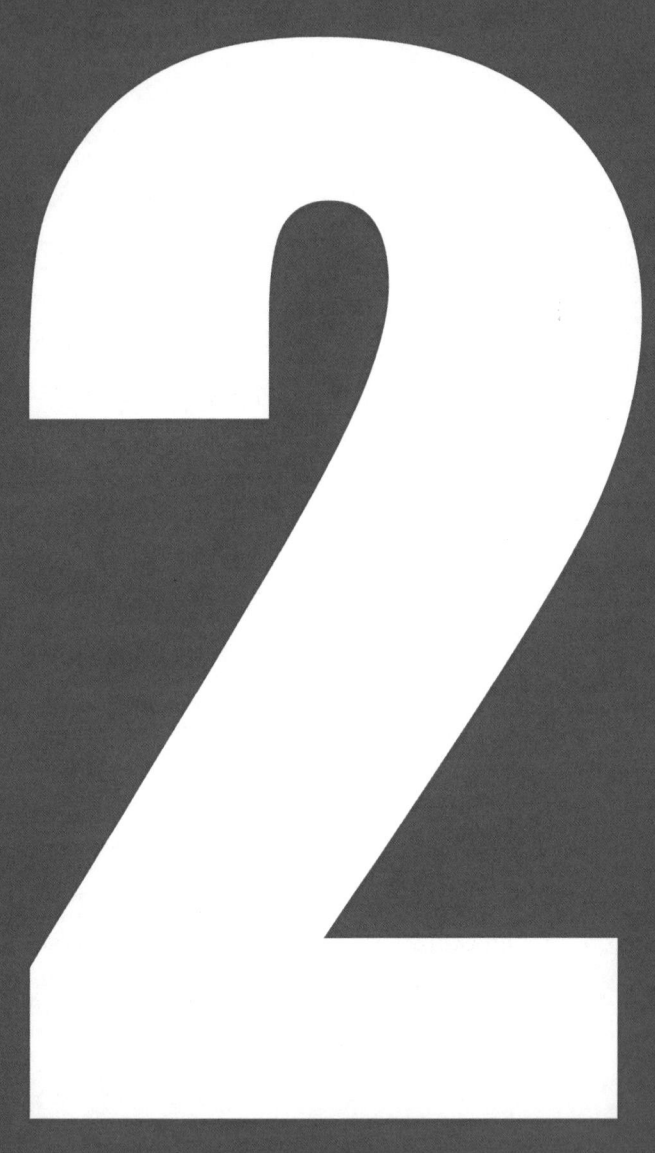

STEP TWO:

COMMUNICATE

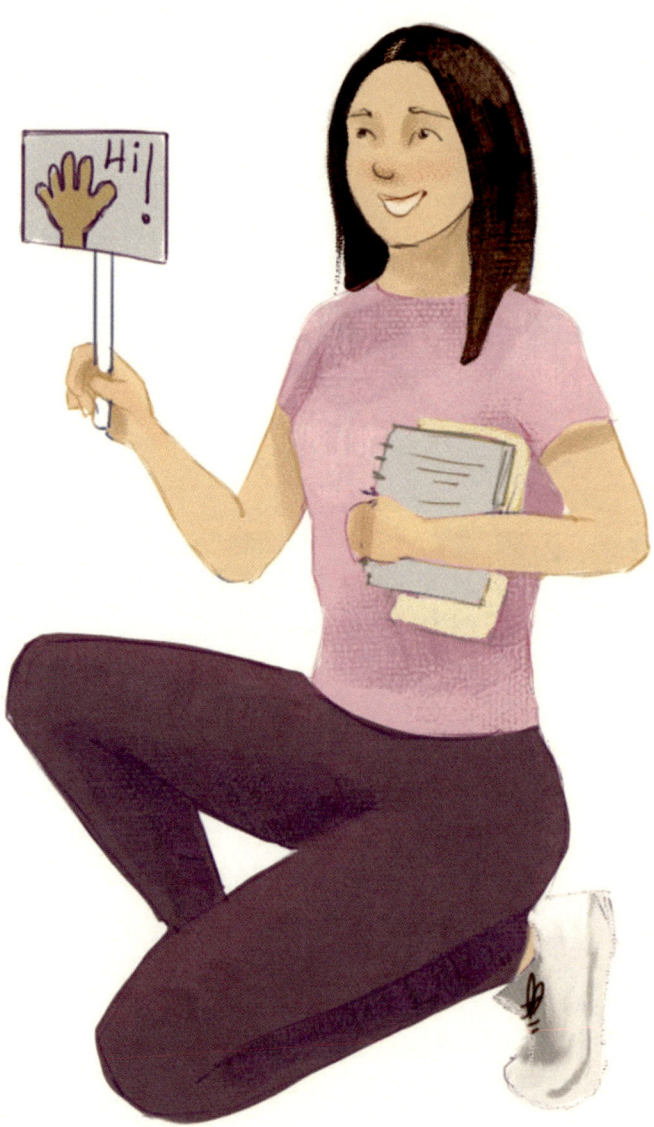

Based on observation, discover the best way to communicate with the child. Watch and listen to his or her words, body language, and how he or she moves and interacts. According to Baniel (2012), when you speak the child's language, you'll notice the child will immediately relax and become more responsive and communicate, maybe even become playful. If you are not speaking the child's language, the child will withdraw or become frustrated. Remember, create a nonthreatening and nonstressful environment vital for skill development (Bompa, 1995).

Communication Application

Blaine was receptive toward play, so play became the focal point to connect best. Sliding a note across the table to open and read immediately communicated playfulness. What was written on the note was a stress-free, friendly invite to play catch. As you can see, play was my common denominator. I knew I was on target by speaking his language once he paused his DS and joined me outside.

3

STEP THREE:

SCHEDULE

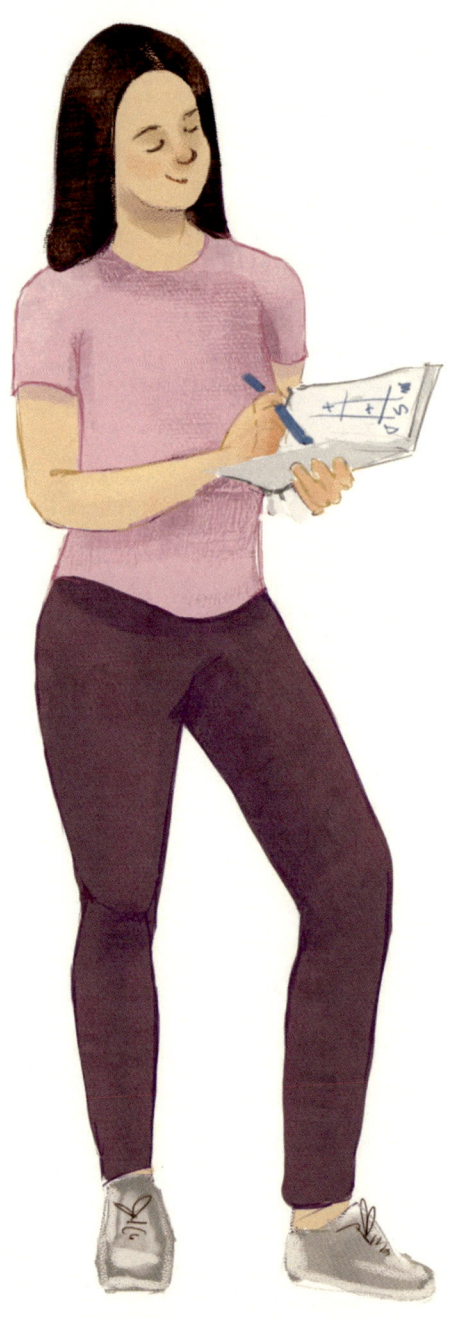

Create a schedule based on the observation and communication vehicles considering age, sensitive periods, demands of sport discipline (if applicable), optimization of the level of physical fitness, the structure of a workout, and gender (Jozef, 1996). Give attention to the order in which you plan exercises. Jozef (1996) recommends special exercises should precede general exercises, speed should precede strength exercises, and strength exercises should precede endurance exercises. Once these structures are prioritized in the schedule, consider inserting rest, play, choice, and free time for a fluid transition between swings of intensity, difficulty, and stimulation to minimize frustration (Jacobs, 2018).

Schedule Application

I like to think of the schedule structures as bricks and the inserts as cement. The inserts are what keep the bricks together to form a solid base—maximizing square footage.

Using Blaine's program as an example to show the relationship between schedule structures and inserts, play initiated our session. Notice how each structure had some element of play. Catch then transitioned to special exercises. Through choice, we transitioned into strength training. Notice how strength training intermittently relied on choice as the intensity increased. Strength training (with choice) transitioned to endurance training (again, with choice). We then transitioned into free time, where he taught me different maneuvers using his DS. Free time served as an opportunity to swap teaching roles (he became the expert; I became the student) and relax before going home. Check out the *Schedule Sample* to see how this looks on paper. The child may prefer using the schedule as a tangible visual, crossing off accomplishments as the session unfolds.

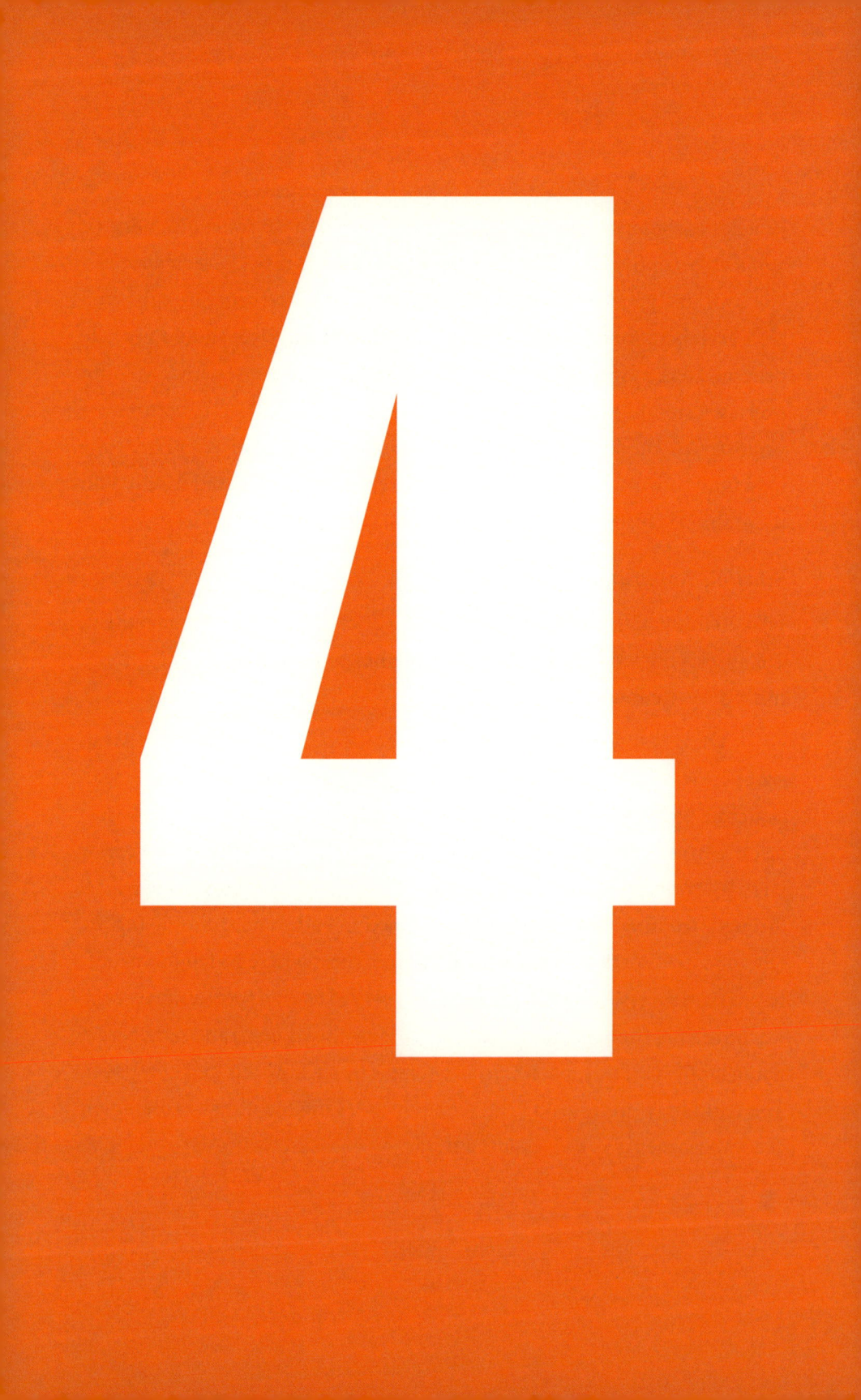

STEP FOUR:

PROGRESS

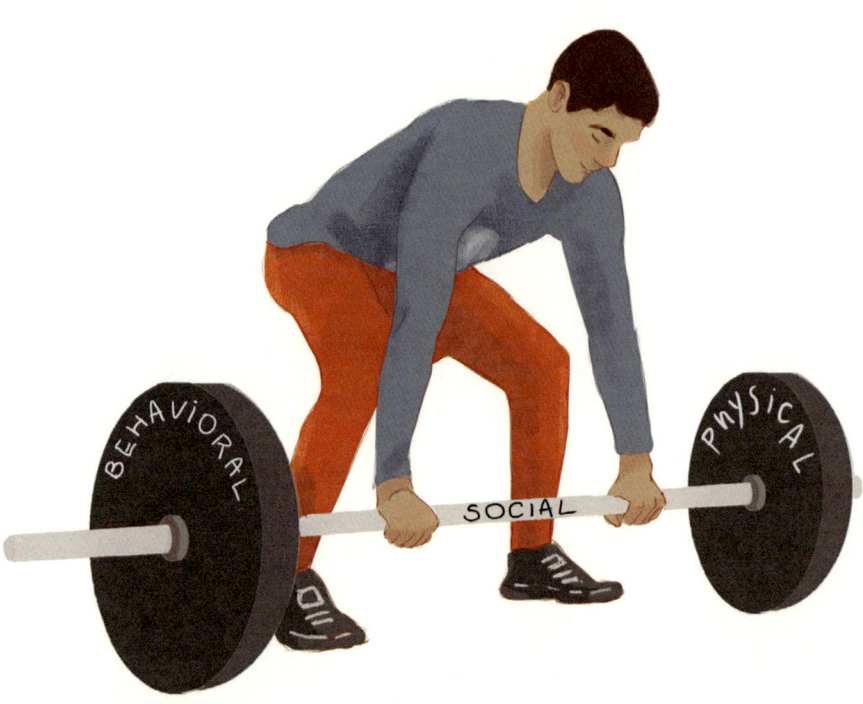

To get a basic progressive training program thriving, delivery, creativity, and patience heavily come into play. Be forewarned, this is commonly where training manuals go wrong, especially when programming for children with autism. Any accredited professional can come up with a detailed and logistical training schedule. Still, how you execute the training program considering physical, behavioral, and social progression is key—this is what separates exercise as a weekend frustration from a lifelong journey.

Realize, although my formal education equipped me with the scholastic and programming know-how, I accredit Anat Baniel for shaping my disposition and fine-tuning my ability to execute instruction properly for children. In her book, *Kids Beyond Limits*, you'll find the nine essentials she uses to maximize child potential through the brain plasticity principles. Through her essentials, my approach and effectiveness working with children with autism transformed, especially in the recreational setting. Think of her nine essentials as the active ingredients in the cement.

In the *Storybook*, the nine essentials repeat and overlap from the observation step to the end of the workout. I urge you to read *Kids Beyond Limits* and begin to apply the essentials.

Physical Progress

According to Jacobs (2018), two or three training sessions should be performed per week. Begin with one per week until two or three training sessions per week is a natural addition for the child. The National Strength and Conditioning Association (2018) recommends a basic progressive resistance training program initiated with one set each of several movements for eight to twelve repetitions and to increase the number of sets per exercise when appropriate. Increases in breathing, sweating, and heart rate should be noticeable. As a reminder, base the order of movements in the schedule per Jozef's recommendations (step three).

Physical Progress Application

As you'll soon come to understand, programming is an art of bridging the gap between theory and practice. In theory, as ideal as it would be to add repetitions, sets, weight, and frequency in a linear fashion, it's unrealistic. In practice, there will be good days, and there will be bad days. Early on, rather than focusing on additions to repetition, set, and weight schemes, consider if the child is having fun, if you're building a relationship with the child, and if the child's technique is slowly looking better. If the child progresses in a small area of their workout, be sure to celebrate. If the child progresses in five areas on a particular day, be sure to celebrate. If the child is on the brink of a meltdown and having a terrible time, shut it down and gladly pick up where you left off another day. Under no circumstances should you communicate to the child that you're let down because your expectations for the day were not met.

Using Blaine's schedule as an example, we tossed the bouncy green ball back and forth in week one until we could no longer successfully make a catch. The game could be played twice after a short rest for week two, assuming his interest remained piqued. As another example, the stability ball kicks for week two could go from five repetitions per variation to six repetitions, with the number of rounds remaining as-is. By week three, it may be acceptable to use a ball smaller in circumference than the stability ball to increase skill difficulty. Again, use your observational skills to judge if the progression will be attainable for the child rather than stress-inducing.

Behavioral Progress

The physical progression should match behavioral strategies to ignite and maintain the child's interest (Jacobs, 2018). Through your communication and schedule vehicles, discover the child's limits to determine why and when meltdowns are likely to erupt to eliminate their occurrence. Therefore, create a messaging system. This system gives the child a manageable way to express a need for rest: time alone, a location change, an intensity drop, a switch in exercise, etc. Here, you're exchanging trust between each other. The child understands you won't dismiss their signal, and you're not perceiving them as whiny or looking to get out of work. This message system also prohibits you from ignoring slight changes in behavior that otherwise, when stacked in accumulation, may lead to disaster.

Behavioral Progress Application

Match current behavioral strategies that are successful in the home and school. If what's in place is not working, create your system. The schedule inserts—rest, play, choice, and free time—help regulate emotion and behavior output as physical demands increase. Through time, watch the reliance on inserts lessen as the child perceives movement as gratifying, enjoyable, and preferable.

Social Progress

Naturally, within the gym setting, a social progression ensues. It begins with the newly formed relationship between the trainer and the child (greatly influenced by parent involvement) and extends to gym members sharing the same space. When appropriate, consider moving from a gym setting to an offsite location for exercise in recreational places of interest. Consider group training. Group training can lead to playdates and social events.

Social Progress Application

Here are eight options for combining fitness and social skills into a designated chunk of time—progressing from *Gym Training* to movement-based playdates. Notice how training types one through eight are rooted in movement, while the comforts of familiarity lead to offsite exploration and social networking.

The starting place is based on the needs of the child. For example, *Gym Training* may be the launch pad, followed by a slow progression to the eighth option, *Playdate with a Friend*. Based on the child's needs, it may be advantageous to pick and choose a training type in an *à la carte* style, providing a new adventure weekly. In the *Storybook*, it was advantageous for Blaine to begin with *Gym Training*. It took a year to get to the point where offsite training became appropriate.

Eight Training Types to Progressively Integrate Social Networks

1. Gym Training

Gym Training takes place in a gym setting. It's a weekly commitment to complete a set of movement-based objectives within a workout at the gym. The primary social connection is the relationship between the trainer and the child.

To smoothly transition from *Gym Training* to *Half Gym–Half Offsite*, train beside other gym members and invite interaction and communication to build associations between exercise and someone other than the trainer. Encourage and model appropriate gym etiquette and social interaction through common courtesy, patience, acknowledgment, conversation, and spatial awareness.

Slowly incorporate new areas to work out within the gym space to communicate that training can be performed at multiple locations with various equipment and people. Consider the parking lot, staircase, gym entrance, cardio room, and powerlifting room as alternatives.

2. Half Gym–Half Offsite

Half Gym–Half Offsite splits a gym session into two halves: one half takes place in the gym; the other half takes place offsite. It's a weekly commitment to complete movement-based objectives in and outside of the gym. The offsite portion gets you out of the gym and places you into a new location that requires physical activity. The location should be near the gym and easily accessible (public and free). It is here that the child will be able to exercise social skills learned in the gym setting, refine, and accumulate more.

In these offsite locations, peer-to-peer interaction is likely. It's an excellent opportunity to introduce social communication and team-building skills when/if appropriate: engaging in conversation, taking turns, winning, losing, leadership, accepting criticism, maintaining a positive attitude, and knowing when to take a break.

Easily accessible locations include a walking/bike trail, public playground, high school track, and public pool. As familiarity occurs by training offsite, slowly add new locations. Begin to lengthen the mileage between the gym and the offsite location.

3. Offsite Training

Offsite Training takes place at an offsite location. It's a weekly commitment to complete movement-based objectives outside of the gym. The location can be nearby or far, but I wouldn't exceed thirty to sixty minutes of driving time. One suggestion is to begin the session at the gym (start with familiarity and review the schedule) and break off from there. You'll have a great opportunity to gauge the child's readiness before venturing into uncharted territory. As you know, some training days should not take place.

Choose movement-based locations to refine previous social and physical lessons and introduce new experiences. In most cases, you'll be surrounded by other individuals looking to have fun while moving—this gives the activity positive exposure and plenty of opportunities to engage and reciprocate with others. These locations tend to be game-like, so this is a great opportunity to develop team-building skills further.

Offsite locations that I recommend are trampoline parks, the zoo, a bowling alley, a public pool, a corn maize farm, and Putt-Putt.

4. Half One-to-One–Half Training Partner

Half One-to-One—Half Training Partner takes place in the gym setting. It's a weekly commitment to complete movement-based objectives inside the gym individually and then with a training partner.

The training partner can be a friend or sibling, someone around the same age with or without autism. In this type of training, we are easing into working with another to complete our workout. The idea is that when the children are together, you're creating an environment that helps both of them work as a unit. Ideally, you'd like to pair two children that physically and socially complement one another by placing them in a situation where they can feed off one another. You will guide this synergistic partnership.

Choose activities that will benefit and provide balance for each child. For example, one child may be very athletic and looking for a challenging and rigid workout, whereas the other child may be looking to have fun with play. Decide how to blend both worlds into one—a world that is productive, worthwhile, and fun.

5. Gym Group Training

Gym Group Training takes place in the gym setting. It's a weekly commitment to complete movement-based objectives inside the gym with one or multiple training partners.

Ideally, this session would begin with the same peer from the previous type of training.

The only difference between this and the last type is now we're ready to complete the entire workout with one or multiple buddies. Similar to *Half One-to-One–Half Training Partner*, the key is creating an environment where everyone thrives for the duration of the session. The union is providing opportunities for each child that would otherwise be nonexistent.

6. Offsite Group Training

Offsite Group Training takes place at an offsite location. It's a weekly commitment to complete movement-based objectives offsite with one or multiple training partners. Choose movement-based locations that will refine previously learned social and physical objectives and introduce new experiences. When planning, consider a meeting place (at the gym or the offsite location) and consider if any help (someone other than you) is necessary.

Although you are familiar with the children and the children are familiar with each other, the dynamics change once the environment changes. Consider planning for unpredictable events and secure extra help. Extra help can always be minimized (if necessary), but without help, you have eliminated possible sources of quick remediation. At first, choose offsite locations with minimal working parts (admission, wait-time, extra space, lots of people, heavy workloads). When comfortable, begin to add more working parts.

7. Home Training

Home Training takes place at home. Despite where this type of training falls numerically, I immediately utilize *Home Training*. At this initial level, *Home Training* involves choosing one familiar exercise or activity/game from *Gym Training* and practicing it at home with a family member. Depending on the needs of the child, this may be a daily or weekly task, sometimes only taking five minutes to complete (including acknowledgment, setup, review of assignment, performance, and tracking). This task is presented as homework and demonstrated for at least one home member to witness expectations. As a reminder, this task is nothing new. It is familiar and easily attainable. One of the most important aspects of this assignment is that you're beginning the transfer process of awareness, practice time, the formation of new habits, changing roles, and taking responsibility.

As number seven on this list, *Home Training* transforms into an entire training session instead of a mini assignment. At this point in the progression, the child is well-versed with training in a group dynamic in various environments. Now at home, this is an excellent opportunity to get the family involved, get creative with indoor and outdoor space, and create new family habits.

8. Playdate with a Friend

Playdate with a Friend is precisely what the title suggests; it's a playdate! It's a weekly or a monthly commitment to have a playdate with a friend, combining movement, personal interest/choice, and fun. *Playdate with a Friend* is a great opportunity to ask where the children would like to go and what they'd like to do. If the children choose the same activity, this is a plus. If the children have different ideas in mind, choose one, then emphasize how you'll do the other activity another time, or combine multiple ideas into one session. For example, complete thirty minutes of batting cages, follow up with an arcade game for fifteen minutes, and finish the session with fifteen minutes of lunch. Note: although the emphasis is on play and freedom, you must provide a framework. What happens within the framework is executed with flexibility and led by the children. Minimize your involvement, if appropriate, and allow the children to take the lead. Playdates naturally reveal child strengths and weaknesses; therefore, use future training sessions as your outlet to strengthen weaknesses noted during the playdate. Now is not the time. Interject if safety is in question. Similar to *Offsite Group Training*, begin these dates with extra hands and eyes and then minimize help when appropriate.

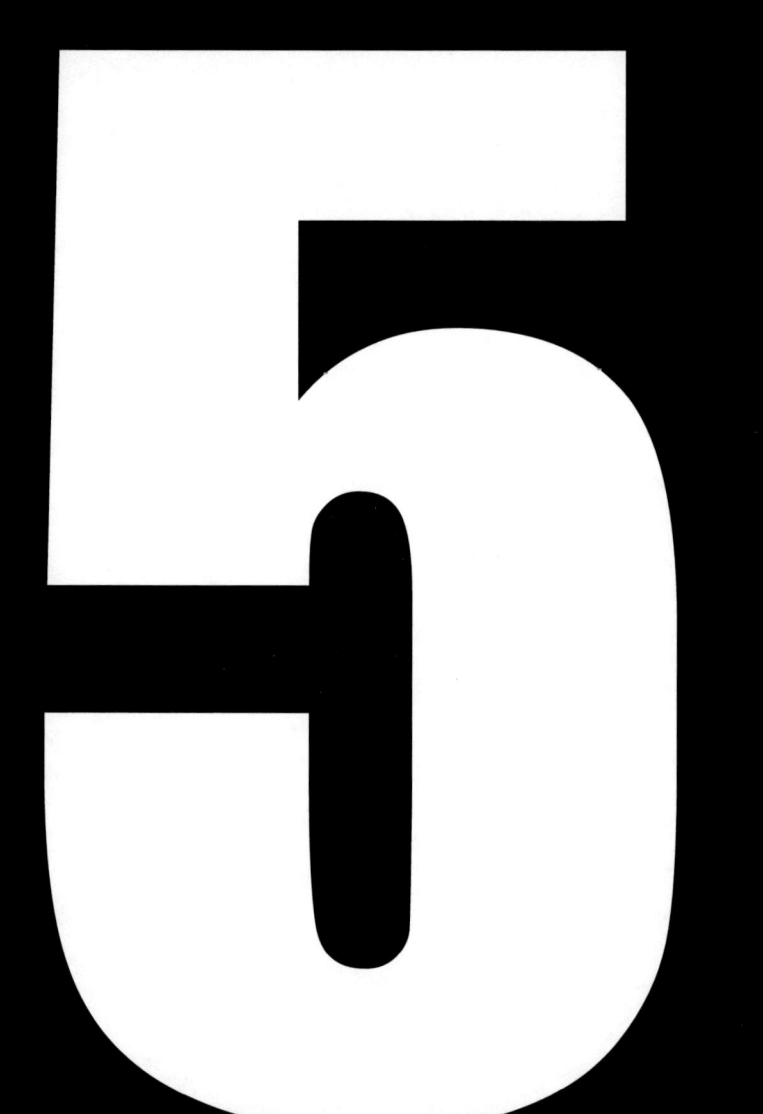

STEP FIVE:

MOTIVATE

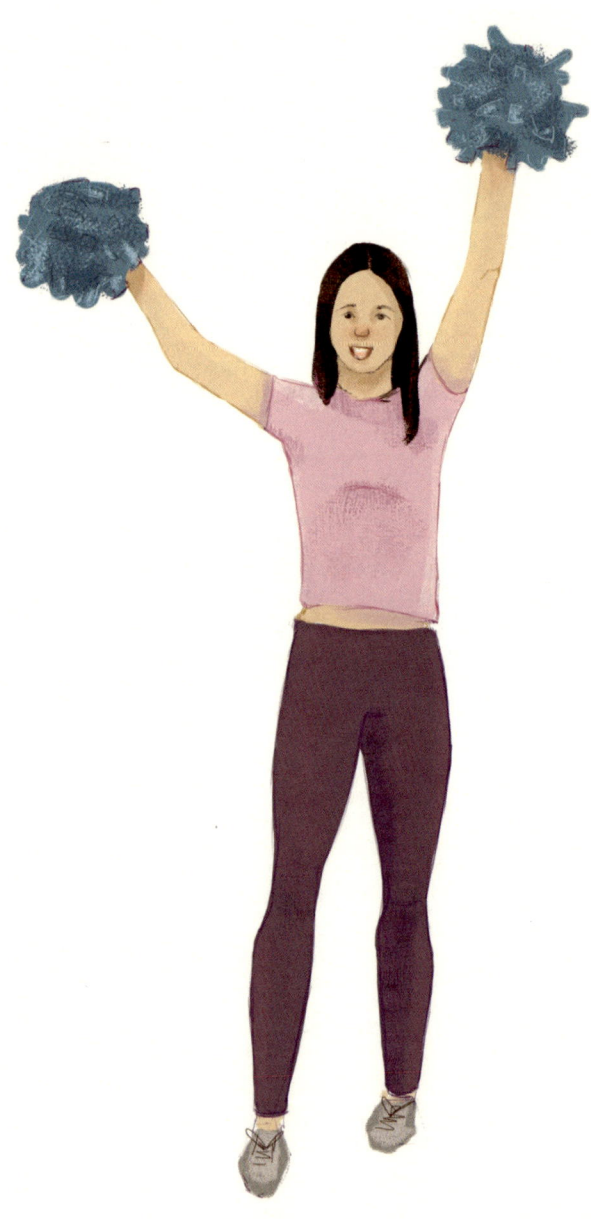

Create a delicate balance between extrinsic and intrinsic motivation when crafting and executing the exercise schedule. Blending the two types of motivation will make the exercise experience meaningful for the child, a place where he or she feels included, curious, in control, and creative (Hinson, 1995). Rely on your observation and communication vehicles to determine what motivators will be unique to the child under your care. You'll be able to fine-tune your motivators as training progresses, and as the needs of the child regularly change.

Extrinsic Motivation Application

Extrinsic rewards are tangible items like certificates, stickers, grades, free time, and food. According to Hinson (1995), it's imperative to avoid using rewards as the focus of the activity. Instead, give rewards independent of the child's expectation.

A preferred extrinsic motivator for Blaine is food from McDonald's. He earns tally marks during training when the effort is high, when he tries new exercises, manipulates new equipment, and does extra work. Once he accumulates twelve tally marks, he earns a meal from McDonald's. After a training session, we'll dine at McDonald's, allowing us to practice restaurant etiquette, make an order, manage money, and enjoy a meal together.

Intrinsic Motivation Application

When children participate in fitness activities for intrinsic reasons, exercise is viewed as a process and not a means to an end. The process leads to personal satisfaction, confidence, and competence. Intrinsically motivating activities have four characteristics in common: challenge, curiosity, control, and creativity (Hinson, 1995). Be sure to handcraft these considerations into every training experience.

Taking a look at Blaine's workout, sliding the note across the table sparked his interest, intriguing him to want to play catch with me. General exercises packaged with play piqued his curiosity, allowing him to take ownership of the session with a sense of control. The workout was challenging based on the new demands impressed upon him (equipment, location, and trainer) and was perceived as not too difficult or too easy. Giving him decision-making power throughout fed his curiosity, creative-thinking skills, and willingness to try new things that would typically frustrate him. Incorporating the four motivating characteristics into our first training session (and every training session thereafter) captivated him enough to come back the following week.

REFERENCES

1. Smith, K. A., Gouze, K. R. (2004). *The Sensory-Sensitive Child*. New York: Harper Collins.

2. Dawson, G., Rosanoff, M. (2009). Sports, Exercise, and the Benefits of Physical Activity for Individuals with Autism. Retrieved from www.autismspeaks.org.

3. Baniel, A. (2012). *Kids Beyond Limits*. New York: Penguin Group.

4. Drabik, J. (1996). *Children & Sports Training*. Vermont: Stadion Publishing Company, Inc.

5. Hillier, A., Murphy, D., Ferrara, C. (2011). A Pilot Study: Short-term Reduction in Salivary Cortisol Following Low Level Physical Exercise and Relaxation among Adolescents and Young Adults on the Autism Spectrum. Retrieved from wileyonlinelibrary.com.

6. Jacobs, P. L. (2018). *NSCA's Essentials of Training Special Populations*. Illinois: Human Kinetics.

7. Bompa, T. (1995). *From Childhood to Champion Athlete*. Canada: Veritas Publishing Inc.

8. Hinson, C. (1995). *Fitness for Children*. Illinois: Human Kinetics.

SCHEDULE SAMPLE

Here is a sixty-minute Schedule Sample based on the illustrated workout from the *Storybook*. Pay attention to the order of operation and the times associated. If appropriate, replicate a tangible schedule (on a piece of paper or dry-erase board) for the child to internalize and manipulate. Create a schedule for personal use to organize your actions and to track progress.

When tracking progress, record weights, repetitions and sets, equipment choices and preferences, duration of the workout, intensity levels, changes in behavior, social skills, celebrations, changes needed, and any other markers that are specific to the child. These notes will better prepare you and the child for the next workout by etching out an appropriate course of action. Decide when it will be appropriate for the child to take ownership of the tracking process and record weights, repetitions, and sets. Reuse the same schedule as interest piques and performance progresses.

1:00–1:05 Hello: Greet and meet with schedule overview

1:05–1:15 Coordination: Stability ball catch (3 rounds) and kicks (3×10)

1:15–1:25 Strength: Stability ball prone walks and static holds (2×8)

1:25–1:35 Game: Hide-n-seek or freeze tag (1 round)

1:35–1:45 Endurance: Obstacle course (2 rounds)

1:45–1:50 Rest

1:50–1:55 Free time: Child's choice

1:55–2:00 Goodbye: Session summary and homework

TRAINING
SUCCESS

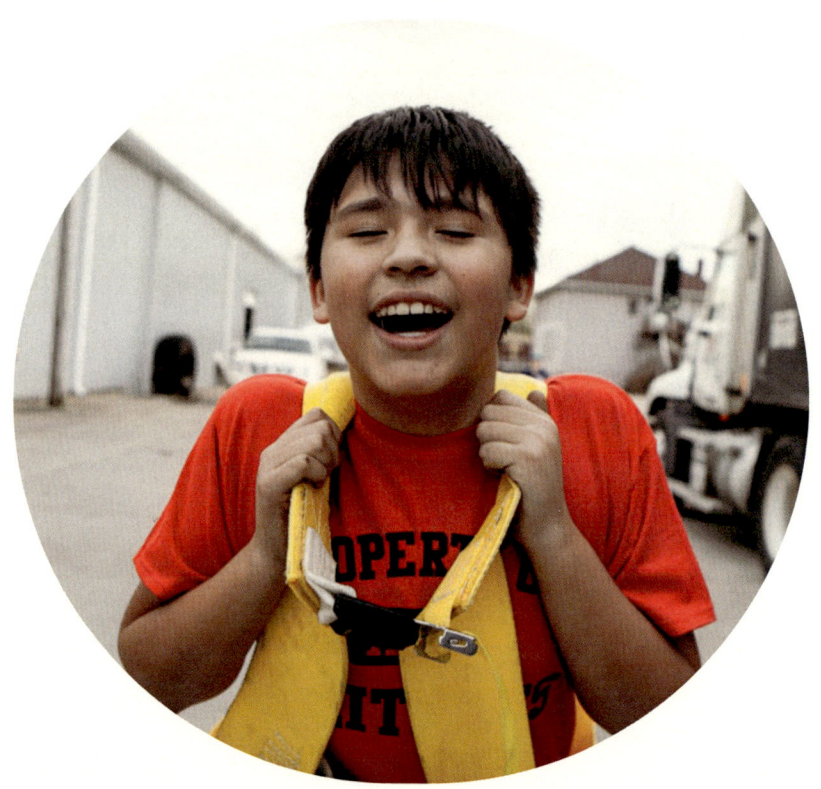

Ken Hicks

In May of 2013, our fitness journey began. Our training schedule has continued weekly since then, roughly three hundred and sixty-four sessions under our belts! In this timeframe, Blaine has gone from weighing one hundred and eighteen pounds as a ten-year-old to two hundred and sixty pounds as a seventeen-year-old, towering six-feet tall. "All muscle," he says. A schedule that was once dependent on play, obstacle courses, and a DS is now dependent on gaining muscle, reaching goals, getting stronger, and working hard. Exercises that once terrified Blaine, like the squat, bench, deadlift, pull-up, jump rope, and box jump, are now part of our weekly regimen. Believe it or not, two years in, I couldn't imagine training outside of the S4 Compound. Yet slowly, Blaine began to gain confidence and competence in his ability to move, which led naturally to offsite training adventures.

For 2021, Blaine will endure another twelve-week training prep to compete in his sixth 5K. Our goal is to beat our previous time and enjoy a day at the zoo.

More than finessing lifting form or adding pounds to the bar and muscle to Blaine's frame, we have created a special bond through training. We're buddies, and we'll continue to use exercise to attain personal records (PRs) inside and outside of the gym for years to come.

PARENTAL FEEDBACK—

WHY THE NOTE IS EMPOWERING

Training has always been an outlet throughout my life—my way to deal with stress, competition, success, failure, anger, and every other emotion known to man.

Raising a son with autism, the gym would serve as his outlet too—his means to develop physically, learn healthy habits, make better choices, be social, and deal with anger and cyclical meltdowns. I mean, it worked for me. Coupling Blaine's familiarity in the gym environment since diapers with my basic physical development know-how, we had some success, but he'd spend most of the time playing video games.

"It worked for me," is one of the worst ideas I've had in my life. It was hard for me because this is what I knew (or at least thought I knew) and could do for my son.

I still remember the day I looked over, and Blaine was not at the table but outside playing ball with Sheena. He was moving! He was laughing! He was having fun! He was exercising!

I won't lie; it was a struggle to train him and a struggle watching someone else train him. What if he had a meltdown? I was the only one who could identify his triggers.

As parents, it's our job to do what is best for our children and what is best for their future—this may not always be aligned with what is best for you or your ego.

What I discovered through Sheena was the process of training—the process is powerful. I was used to training progressions, but what Blaine needed was what I would best describe as regressions, a lower starting point with the integration of research-based teaching strategies and common sense.

"Do you want to play catch?"

Simple.

Empowering.

The Power of a Note is the story of how one note can make a world of difference.

Dave Tate, BS, CSCS

CEO, elitefts.com Inc.

AUTHOR BIO

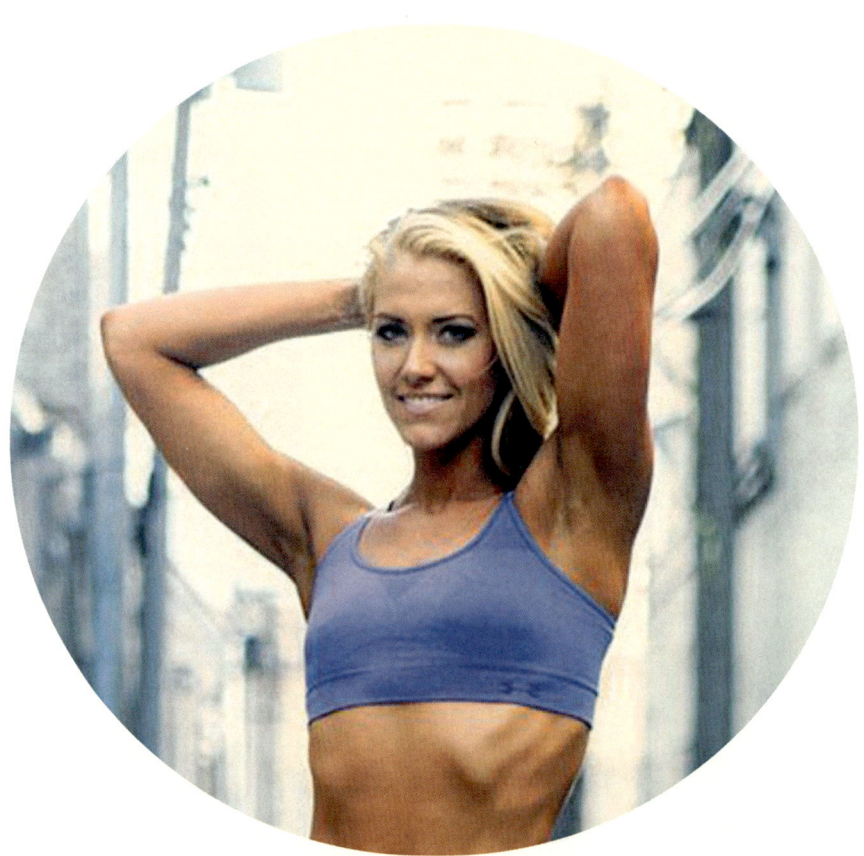

Pat Lee

Sheena Leedham earned her master's degree in education at Edinboro University with a concentration in elementary education and recreation administration. Her educational background led her to specialize in programming for children and adults with autism in the public school setting, a partial hospitalization program, Barber National Institute, a private gym setting, Turning Pointe Autism Foundation, and Ohio State University. Through the Ohio State University's Nisonger Center, Sheena coordinates a social support group event every month for teens and young adults with autism to experience the Greater Columbus Area. Sheena also consults Ohio State University's ACE! and PLAN programs, where she creates a physical and nutritional curriculum to educate autistic high school and college students on the importance of habitual fitness and proper nutrition. You can find her special needs column at *www.elitefts.com*, where she educates families and trainers on why and how to incorporate movement into the lives of children with autism—it's here that you'll find the training progress of Blaine, too.